IMPROVING MOBILITY IN OLDER PERSONS

A Manual for Geriatric Specialists

Carole B. Lewis, Ph.D.

Physical Therapy Services
Washington, D.C.

Aspen Series in Physical Therapy

Carole B. Lewis
Series Editor

AN ASPEN PUBLICATION®
Aspen Publishers, Inc.
Gaithersburg, Maryland
1989

The authors have made every effort to ensure the accuracy of the information herein. However, appropriate information sources should be consulted, especially for new or unfamiliar procedures. It is the responsibility of every practitioner to evaluate the appropriateness of a particular opinion in the context of actual clinical situations and with due consideration to new developments. Authors, editors, and the publisher cannot be held responsible for any typographical or other errors found in this book.

Library of Congress Cataloging-in-Publication Data

Lewis, Carole Bernstein.
Improving mobility in older persons: a manual for geriatric specialists/Carole Lewis.
p. cm.
"An Aspen publication."
Includes bibliographies and index.
ISBN: 0-8342-0020-1
1. Physical therapy for the aged. I. Title.
[DNLM: 1. Gait--in old age. 2. Locomotion--in old age. 3. Posture--in old age. WT 104 L673i]
RC953.8.P58L48   1988   615.8′2′0880565--dc19   DNLM/DLC
for Library of Congress
88-24244
CIP

Editorial Services: Mary Beth Roesser

Library of Congress Catalog Card Number: 88-24244
ISBN: 0-8342-0020-1

Printed in the United States of America

3 4 5

Dedication

I dedicate this book to my adorable, loving husband, Mark. Before I met Mark, whenever I lectured on aging, I would show a videotape about a woman with Alzheimer's disease entitled "Living with Grace." This film depicts Grace's husband as an unbelievably understanding, patient, and loving spouse. I would joke with my students, saying that if they ever found anyone like that, I was single and lived in Washington, D.C. Now I don't need their help because I have found someone with those qualities.

Thank you, Mark, for supporting and loving me throughout the writing of this book and throughout our lives.

Table of Contents

Preface

This book is written from the perspective of a therapist who sees older patients every day in various settings. It is a base from which all therapists can begin to create new ideas, research, and clinical directions. This base will provide the proper perspective from which to view the treatment of older persons.

My recent work has been in the area of clinical practice as well as reimbursement for this practice. The reimbursement issue is an underlying motive for writing this book, which describes how to improve patient care through obtaining reimbursement.

One of the main ideas that became apparent to me while working on reimbursement and proper documentation was that there was no common thread among therapists regarding evaluation and treatment. Patients were not receiving enough care because there was no way to ensure reimbursement. It is my hope that by quantifying the way in which therapists treat their patients, reimbursement will be improved.

This book identifies some nonabsolute but reproducible scales that can be used for various disabilities and impairments experienced by the older person. These scales measure functional deficits from transfers all the way up to high-level walking and screening for balance problems.

My hope is that, when reading this book, specialists will be able to integrate many of the ideas quantified in these scales into a system of physical therapy that works for them.

I have tried to avoid subjects with which many therapists are already familiar. These topics, treatment of pressure sores, drug interactions, and balance exercises, are, however, discussed in the appendixes.

The discussions in the book parallel the treatment priorities for the mobility spectrum so that specialists can use the manual to find evaluation forms for specific problems and use them sequentially. If a specialist is having difficulty with one aspect of treatment, such as transfers, and wants to evaluate the range of motion of the patient's hips in the standing portion of transfer, he or she can quickly look to the transfer section and find the appropriate scales and discussion. The specialist can also read discussions of greater detail in each section.

In addition, I believe this book can be easily read and gives a sense of continuity between sections. Many times we lose sight of the direction taken in patient treatment, but it is important to keep on course. It has been my focus in writing this book to develop a system to help therapists maintain a systematic approach.

I hope that this book will aid in evaluations and treatment and in the focusing and directing of treatment strategy. I also hope that each reader enjoys the book and will use it to help older patients achieve or maintain good health and to appreciate life to the fullest.

Acknowledgments

I thank Margaret Quinlin for being a great editor and friend. I also thank Margaret Langdon for being such a delightful model and patient.

The Mobility Spectrum

The average life expectancy of a person in the United States has increased from approximately 50 years at the beginning of the 19th century to 74 years in 1980.[1] Because of the added years of activity, older persons are experiencing more wear and tear on the body, and this affects their mobility. The health care team needs to look at ways to compensate for the wear and tear so that older people can remain mobile and independent as long as possible. Many problems in mobility cannot be cured with a pill or by surgical intervention; they can be resolved only by a slow, gradual rehabilitation process. The investment of time, effort, and expertise required is worth it, however, to achieve optimal function in aging individuals and improve their quality of life.

The term *dysmobility* denotes any problem related to getting from one place to another. Such problems range from difficulties in getting in and out of bed to difficulties in rolling in bed, standing, transferring from bed to bath, driving a car, walking along a street, or going up and down stairs.

The mobility spectrum ranges from optimal functioning to total dependence (Figure 1-1). Along the mobility spectrum there are degrees of optimal functioning or dependence in bed mobility, sitting, transfers, standing, ambulating, and balancing. In addition, balance is also intimately woven throughout all the upright postures. Cardiopulmonary, musculoskeletal, neurological, sensory, and psychological variables all play significant roles in each of the aspects of the mobility spectrum. This is the framework for working with the older population on independent function.

Health care professionals need to realize that there is a spectrum for mobility and that older people can enjoy optimal functioning at any level of the mobility spectrum. The goal is to help them achieve their highest possible function in each level of the spectrum. That may mean, for exam-

Figure 1-1 Mobility Spectrum

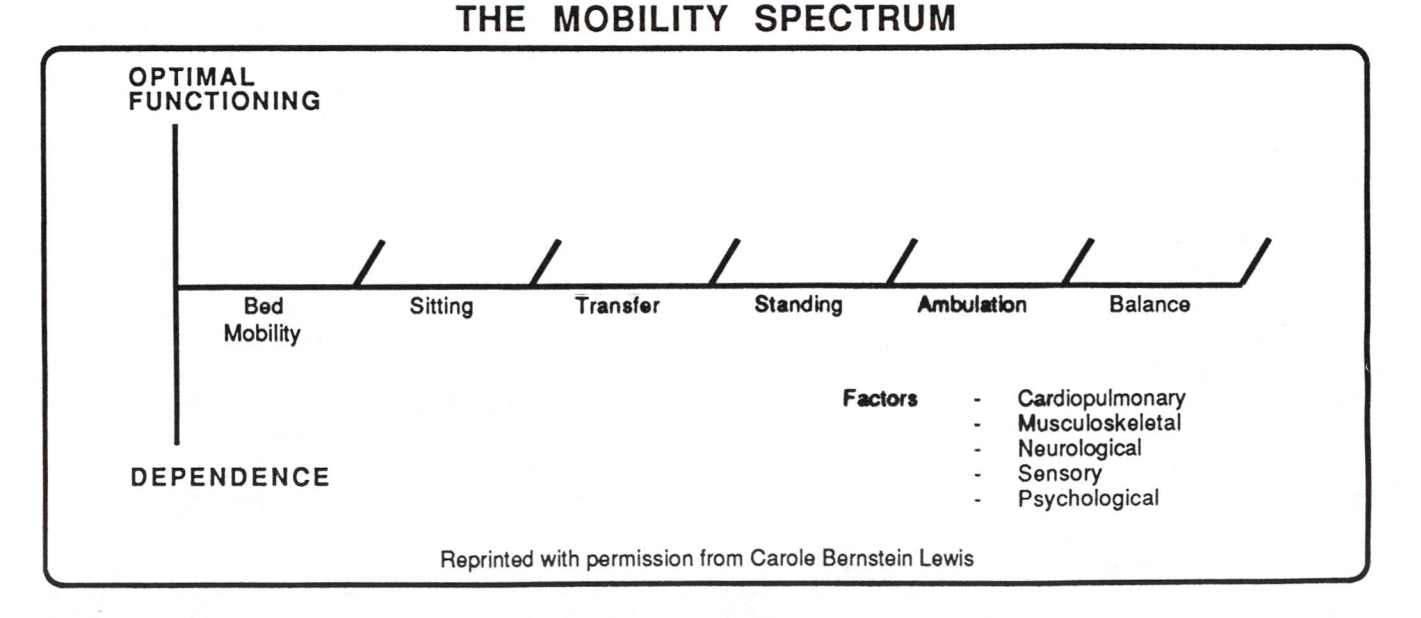

THE MOBILITY SPECTRUM

OPTIMAL
FUNCTIONING

Bed Mobility   Sitting   Transfer   Standing   Ambulation   Balance

Factors - Cardiopulmonary
 - Musculoskeletal
 - Neurological
 - Sensory
 - Psychological

DEPENDENCE

Reprinted with permission from Carole Bernstein Lewis

ple, teaching a wheelchair-bound person to get in and out of the wheelchair independently and without fear. On the other hand, it may mean working on balance with someone who walks 4 miles a day and has recently become fearful of falling.

Dysmobility risks for older persons arise throughout the mobility spectrum. Older persons at the very extreme ends of the mobility spectrum have the greatest risk for falling; those people who transfer from bed to wheelchair are at very high risk, and those who walk a great deal are also at high risk.[2] The greater the person's activity, the greater the person's chance of falling.[3] Therefore, health care professionals may want to use just this one piece of data to begin investigating the ends of the spectrum for improving older persons' mobility. Rehabilitation will then become less myopic and will stop being focused only on walking or gait training.

OLDER POPULATION

An examination of the background information on the older population in the United States re-vealed that this segment of the population has grown tremendously. In 1900, people over 65 made up 5 percent of the U.S. population; in 1985 they made up 11.8 percent.[4] Moreover, there were 17 million older women and 11.5 million older men in 1985.[5] This difference between the number of men and the number of women affects the support systems that help people remain independent. For example, the husband-wife system may be an unrealistic option in later life. Thus, rehabilitation specialists must use their imagination to provide support systems.

In addition, the older population is getting older. There has been a large increase in the number of "old, old" people (over the age of 85), and these people have more disabilities.[6] Figure 1-2 shows additional statistics on the older population.

Community surveys of the elderly revealed that 15 percent of the population over 65 years of age have some type of mobility problem.[7] In addition, almost 85 percent of people confined to nursing homes have some major problem with mobility.[8] These are rather striking findings in view of the fact that elderly people tend to underreport mobility problems.

Figure 1-2 Facts About Older People. *Source*: Copyright 1988 American Association of Retired Persons. Reprinted with permission.

The Older Population

■ The older population—persons 65 years or older—numbered 28.5 million in 1985. They represented 12.0% of the U.S. population, about one in every eight Americans. The number of older Americans increased by 2.8 million or 11% since 1980, compared to an increase of 4% for the under-65 population.

■ In 1985, there were 17.0 million older women and 11.5 million older men, or a sex ratio of 147 women for every 100 men. The sex ratio increased with age, ranging from 122 for the 65-69 group to a high of 251 for persons 85 and older.

■ The older population itself is getting older. In 1985 the 65-74 age group (17.0 million) was nearly eight times larger than in 1900, but the 75-84 group (8.8 million) was 11 times larger and the 85+ group (2.7 million) was 22 times larger.

■ In 1985, persons reaching age 65 had an average life expectancy of an additional 16.8 years (18.6 years for females and 14.6 years for males).

■ About 2.1 million persons celebrated their 65th birthday in 1985 (5,600 per day). In the same year, about 1.5 million persons 65 or older died, resulting in a net increase of over 560,000 (1,540 per day).

Future Growth

■ The older population is expected to continue to grow in the future (see fig. 1). This growth will slow somewhat during the 1990's because of the relatively small number of babies born during the Great Depression of the 1930's. The most rapid increase is expected between the years 2010 and 2030 when the "baby boom" generation reaches age 65.

■ By 2030, there will be about 65 million older persons, 2 and one-half times their number in 1980. If current fertility and immigration levels remain stable, the only age groups to experience significant growth in the next century will be those past age 55.

■ By the year 2000, persons 65+ are expected to represent 13.0% of the population, and this percentage may climb to 21.2% by 2030.

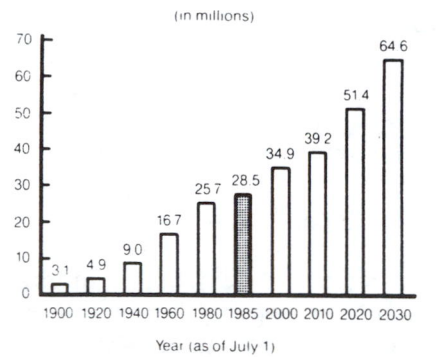

NUMBER OF PERSONS 65+: 1900 to 2030

(in millions)

Year (as of July 1)

Note: Increments in years on horizontal scale are uneven.
Based on data from U S Bureau of the Census

FROM: A Profile of Older Americans, 1986 American Association of Retired Persons, Washington, D.C., 1986

SYSTEMIC CAUSES OF DYSMOBILITY

Musculoskeletal disorders, particularly arthritis, are significant causes of mobility problems in the elderly. Age-related changes in the musculoskeletal system may impact mobility. The cross linking of collagen can cause stiffness to occur more quickly and easily in muscles, fascia, ligaments, joint capsules, and tendons. A decreasing activity level also contributes to decreased muscle and bone strength. Arthritis affects 50 percent of the people over the age of 65 and 75 percent of the people over the age of 80.[9] Arthritis can cause pain, stiffness, swelling, and weakness, all of which affect the ease and efficiency of movement. In addition to arthritis and other musculoskeletal diseases (e.g., osteoporosis and Paget's disease), fractures and problems with the feet commonly occur in older people; obviously these conditions also affect mobility.

The age-related neurological changes that occur with age include:

- decreased proprioception of toes and feet
- increased sway
- increased reaction time
- decreased sense of vibration at the ankles
- decreased number of neurons
- decreased cerebral blood flow
- increased cerebrovascular resistance.[10–12]

Neurological conditions such as stroke, Parkinson's disease, and peripheral neuropathies also increase in prevalence with age. Any of these pathologies may not only themselves affect a person's mobility but may also compound the normal neurological changes that occur with age and thus increase the impact of normal changes on a person's mobility.

Cardiopulmonary problems that sometimes develop with age can also complicate mobility. Changes in the cardiopulmonary system can affect the heart's efficiency in the delivery of nutrients to muscles, nerves, and bones. In addition, the homeostatic mechanisms regulated by the heart may become less effective. If, as a result, the brain and muscles do not receive oxygen and blood in a timely fashion, balance and coordination problems may develop. Pathological problems, such as congestive heart failure, coronary artery disease, emphysema, and peripheral vascular disease, exacerbate normal cardiopulmonary changes and can affect a person's mobility.

Finally, sensory factors (e.g., presbyopia and presbycusis) and psychological factors play a role in the older person's ability to move around. Rehabilitation specialists must become sensitive to all of the systemic complications of mobility.

HISTORY AND GOAL SETTING

Once the causes of dysmobility have been determined, the rehabilitation specialist should take a thorough history that includes:

- the activities the patient has been doing
- the activities the patient would like to do but cannot do
- the length of time the patient has had the problem

- the adaptions the patient has made in the environment and in the daily schedule to work within the dysmobility.

It is very important not only to ask how long the patient has had the problem but to probe for additional information. For example, the rehabilitation specialist should try to find out how the patient is adapting to the problem because the method of adaption may be increasing the dysmobility. For example, the person may be bending forward more in the neck area because it "feels" better. This forward hunched posture can overstretch the tissues originally causing the problem and thus make the problem worse. Exhibit 1–1 lists sample history questions.

Once the history has been established, it is time to set goals with the patient. Goals should include both short-term goals for one to three weeks and long-term goals ranging from six weeks to one year or longer. When working with patients who have had a dysmobility problem for a long time, the rehabilitation specialist should make sure that these patients are aware of the extended period of

Exhibit 1-1 History Questions

1. When did your problem begin?
2. How long have you had this problem?
3. What types of activities were you doing prior to this?
4. What activities are you doing now?
5. What would you like to be doing?
6. How have you changed your life or surroundings to do what you are doing?
   - Are you using family or friends more?
   - Are you using a cane or walker?
   - Are you holding on to furniture more frequently?
   - Are you less active or sleeping longer?

time that is necessary to get results. (One year is a good average.) Patients must commit themselves to one year of serious effort: doing exercises and becoming sensitive to the various aspects of physical functioning so that they can become more in tune with their body. In the meantime, however, they can work on short-term, attainable goals. For a patient who has had a stroke and is having a difficult time sitting up but who wants to be independent, the short-term goal may be improvement in sitting strength, balance, and tolerance; the long-term goal may be independence in transfers so that the patient does not need any family assistance to carry out daily activities.

In each treatment session, it is extremely important to help patients feel that they are achieving improvement along the mobility spectrum, e.g., showing a patient the comparison of his or her heart rate initially to the heart rate today or keeping a permanent record of the person's step length on shelf paper and comparing this on a monthly basis with the patient. Once the history and goals have been established, the rehabilitation specialist can begin to consider assessment and treatment along the mobility spectrum.

To conclude, an allusion to one more concept is necessary. The concept is optimal health. Roger's Health Status Scale[13] (see Figure 1-3) illustrates this. The first category, optimal health, is viewed as a state of complete physical, psychological, and social well-being. The state of suboptimal health is viewed as appearing normal but having possible

Figure 1-3 Health Status Scale. *Source*: Adapted with permission of Macmillan Publishing Company from *Human Ecology and Health Introduction* by Edward S. Rogers. Copyright © 1960 by Edward S. Rogers.

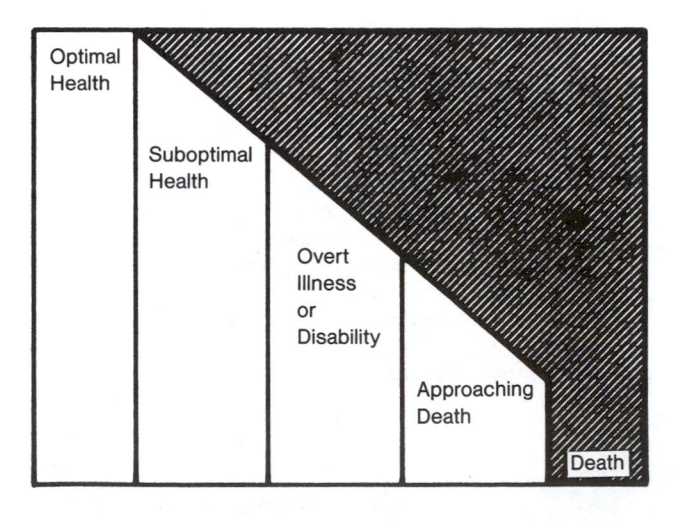

nutritional and physical deficits that may require deeper investigation. An example of this may be a 70-year-old woman with undetected osteoporosis. Overt illness, approaching death, and death are the remaining categories of health status and the main areas for care in the traditional medical model. This book gives ideas and suggestions for treating patients and clients in the area of suboptimal health with goals of reaching optimal health.

An example illustrates this objective: If a 70-year-old woman has undetected osteoporosis, she classically will have to fall and break a hip before she will be seen by rehabilitation specialists. However, she should receive a falls screening to assess problems and to keep her from falling. This look at preventive measures can be used all the way along the mobility spectrum from preventing pressure sores to preventing falls. Not only does this preventive approach have the potential to decrease the overuse of traditional medical intervention, it also has the potential to improve the quality of life for older patients by helping them achieve optimal health.

NOTES

1. "The Aging Population," *P.T. Bulletin,* 1, no. 4 (1987): 2.
2. S. Baker and A. Harvey, "Fall Injuries in the Elderly," *Clinics in Geriatric Medicine* 1 (1985): 501.
3. R. La Porte and R. Sandler, "Physical Activity and Osteoporosis" (Paper presented at the National Institute on Aging Consensus Development Conference, Washington, D.C., April 1984).
4. R. Weg, *The Aged: Who, Where, How-Well* (Los Angeles: Ethel Percy Andrews Gerontology Center, 1979).
5. Ibid.
6. Ibid.
7. Ibid.
8. Ibid.
9. G.P. Rodman, C. McEwen, and S.L. Wallace, *Primer on the Rheumatic Diseases.* Reprinted from *The Journal of the American Medical Association* 224, no. 5 (April 30, 1973) (Supplement).
10. C. Berg, "The Aging Brain," in Strong, W. Wood and Burke, eds., *Central Nervous System Disorders of Aging* (New York: Raven Press, 1988), pp. 7–25.
11. R. Katzman and R.D. Terry, "Normal Aging of the Nervous System," in R. Katzman and R.D. Terry, eds., *The Neurology of Aging* (Philadelphia: F.A. Davis Co., 1983), p. 15.
12. A.R. Patvin et al., "Human Neurologic Function and the Aging Process," *Journal of the American Geriatric Society* 28 (1980): 1.
13. M. Lee and M. Itoh, "The Epidemiology of Disability as Related to Rehabilitation," in Krusen and Kotke, eds., *Handbook of Physical Medicine and Rehabilitation* (Philadelphia: W.B. Saunders, 1971), pp. 879–897.

Bed Mobility

II

The first stage of the mobility spectrum is bed mobility, which is simply the efficiency and the effectiveness with which a person maneuvers in bed. For someone who only sleeps in a bed, bed mobility competence has a less significant value than it has for patients who spend all their time in bed. The assessment of bed mobility involves two distinct areas: immobility and activity.

BED MOBILITY

Bed rest has adverse effects on several body systems (Table 2–1), and these effects lead to many of the complaints commonly heard from older people. If a person is immobile in bed, an assessment of the person's susceptibility to the life-threatening complications of immobility (e.g., cardiovascular deconditioning and pressure sores) must be a part of the rehabilitation effort.

Cardiovascular Deconditioning

Even in young people, cardiovascular conditioning decreases after 48 hours of bed rest.[1] It continues to decline as bed rest continues. Cardiovascular deconditioning can lead to drastic changes in the body; the treatment is to get the person up and moving around.

The longer the person stays in bed, the more difficult each step along the mobility spectrum will be. For example, sitting up for 20 minutes may be as stressful for an older person who has been on bed rest as running 2 miles is for a 40-year-old. Therefore, the rehabilitation specialist should not only encourage activity but should carefully monitor cardiovascular parameters while the patient is progressing along the mobility spectrum (e.g., check heart rate and blood pressure every five minutes for severely deconditioned patients). The activities that the rehabilitation team works on with

Table 2-1 Adverse Effects of Bed Rest

Effects	*Care Indicated*
Musculoskeletal Function	
• Muscular atrophy	Early bed activities that require the patient to use own remaining muscle power
• Osteoporosis	Stress on skeletal system
• Joint stiffness	Range of motion exercises
Cardiovascular Function	
• Thrombus	Proper and frequent positioning
• Edema	Gentle movement exercises to swollen areas
• 30% harder on the heart	Early mobilization
• Orthostatic hypotension	Up as soon as possible
Respiratory Function	
• Status of secretions	Turning, coughing, and deep breathing
• Respiration slower and more shallow	As much activity as possible
• Hypostatic pneumonia	Activity, coughing, and deep breathing
Gastrointestinal Function	
• Constipation	Early mobilization, exercise, and bed activities
• Fecal impaction	Adequate fluids, up as soon as possible
• Negative nitrogen balance	Proper diet

Genitourinary Function
- Urinary status
- Infections

Stress on skeletal system activities
Change in position, forced fluids (300 ml/day)

Decubitus Ulcers

Frequent and proper positioning according to individual skin tolerance

Metabolic Effects
- Dilated blood vessels
- Increased heat
- Increased sweating
- Loss of electrolytes
- Increase in urinary excretion

Up as much as possible
Sitting in chair
Minimal bed clothes
Forced fluids
High protein diet

Psychological Effects
- Decreased sensory stimulation
- Perception of body image altered
- Perception of sensations that do not exist
- Altered perception of existing sensory stimulation
- Increased dependence

Provision of concrete and real environmental stimulations (e.g., clock, calendar, television, radio); observation of activities; extension of environment beyond room and bed (e.g., view through window)
Promotion of independence

the patient should be specific for the functional goals because activities that are focused on the specific goals do not waste the older person's precious and scarce energy.

Pressure Sores

Although pressure sores can occur in patients who sit up, they usually occur in bedridden patients. According to Shepard, Parker, and De-Clucque,[2] pressure sores are seen in an average of 3 to 24 percent of the patients who are admitted to nursing homes. Miller and Elliott[3] found that 64 percent of nursing home patients with pressure sores already had these sores when they were admitted to the nursing home. This finding suggests that hospitals need to place a greater emphasis on the prevention of pressure sores. Once a pressure sore has developed, it can increase the cost of care up to 50 percent[4] because the patients require additional medication, nursing attention, and medical attention until the sore is healed, which can take a long time.

A pressure sore is a significant complication of immobility. When people do not move, certain areas of the body come under more pressure than the skin can normally sustain, pressure is sustained for an extended time, and the tissue dies because of a lack of nutrients. This can happen even when the skin is normal. These sores must be taken into account in rehabilitation plans.

The patients most at risk for pressure sores are those who:

- have lost both sensation and mobility (e.g., patients with multiple sclerosis and paraplegic patients)

- have lost sensation only (e.g., patients with peripheral neuropathies)

- have lost mobility only (e.g., patients with Parkinson's disease)

- are unconscious (e.g., comatose patients)

- are unwilling to move (e.g., patients with arthritis or postoperative pain).

The key to treating people with pressure sores is to screen them, get them up, and get them moving.

One method of screening is the use of the Modified Norton Scale (Exhibit 2–1).[5] In order to use this scale, the rehabilitation specialist simply exercises professional judgment to choose the appropriate ranking for the patient under each of five categories:

1. general physical conditioning
2. mental status
3. activity
4. mobility
5. incontinence

Once the rankings have been chosen, the scores are added. Patients with a score from 17 to 20 are generally healthy and active and at very low risk for developing pressure sores. Patients with a score of 14 or below are considered at high risk for developing pressure sores, and patients with a score of less than 12.9 have a 96 percent chance of developing pressure sores. Furthermore, those with a score of 12 or under have a 51 percent chance of developing pressure sores within two weeks.[6]

Prevention of pressure sores is more cost-effective than is treatment. The best approach to prevention is movement that varies body positions and takes the pressure off those areas where pressure sores may develop. A formal turning schedule may facilitate the prevention of pressure sores (Table 2–2). When a pressure sore does occur, treatment consists of taking pressure off the area and allowing the sore to heal. Appendix A is an issue of *Focus on Geriatric Care & Rehabilitation* specifically on the topic of pressure sores that was written to stimulate thoughts on ways to prevent and treat pressure sores creatively.[7]

Positioning for Comfort and Function

Positioning to avoid pressure sores is crucial; however, when patients are in pain, positioning for function and comfort is also important for rehabilitation success. Rehabilitation specialists should use pillows to enhance comfort without encouraging positions that will cause stiffness and tight muscles (Figure 2-1). To achieve a prone position in patients with hip flex or tightness, progressive positioning is helpful (Figure 2–2).

Exhibit 2-1 Modified Norton Scale

Name _____

Diagnosis _____

Functional Problems _____

A	B	C	D	E
General Physical Condition	Mental Status	Activity	Mobility	Incontinence
4. Good	4. Alert	4. Ambulates	4. Full Motion	4. None
3. Fair	3. Apathetic	3. Walks With Help	3. Slightly Limited	3. Occasional
2. Poor	2. Confused	2. Chair Bound	2. Very Limited	2. Usually/urine
1. Very Bad	1. Stupor	1. Bed	1. Immobile	1. Doubly

Date	A	B	C	D	E	Preventive and Therapeutic Measures

Source: Adapted from *Journal of Enterostomal Therapy,* Vol. 13, pp. 13–38, with permission of The C.V. Mosby Company, © 1986.

Table 2-2 Turning Schedule: Sample Positioning Schedule for Patients on Complete Bed Rest

Time	Position	Activity
6 AM–8 AM	Left sidelying	Breakfast: feeds self; bowel program every other day
8 AM–10 AM	Supine	Bed bath, including range of motion
10 AM–11 AM	Prone	Back care, work up tolerance to 40 min (turn to right)
11 AM–1 PM	Right sidelying	Lunch: feeds self
1 PM–3 PM	Left sidelying	Visiting
3 PM–4 PM	Prone	Back; range of motion; tolerates 40 min, try increase (turn to supine)
6 PM–8 PM	Right sidelying	Dinner: feeds self; visiting
8 PM–11 PM	Left sidelying	Evening care
11 PM–3 AM	Supine	Sleeping
3 PM–6 AM	Right sidelying	Sleeping

Source: Reprinted from *Basic Rehabilitation Techniques: A Self-Instructional Guide,* 3rd ed., by R.D. Sine et al., p. 52, Aspen Publishers, Inc., © 1988.

BED ACTIVITY

The short-term rehabilitation goal for a person who is immobile is to get the person moving in bed. The rehabilitation specialist should help the patient to move sideways, to roll from supine to prone, and to roll over. This activity not only increases movement but also improves cardiovascular response.

People use the various segments of their body differently. In a study conducted at St. Louis University to explore bed activities, Richter[8] identified different movement patterns that people use to roll

Figure 2-1 Positioning for Comfort

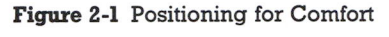

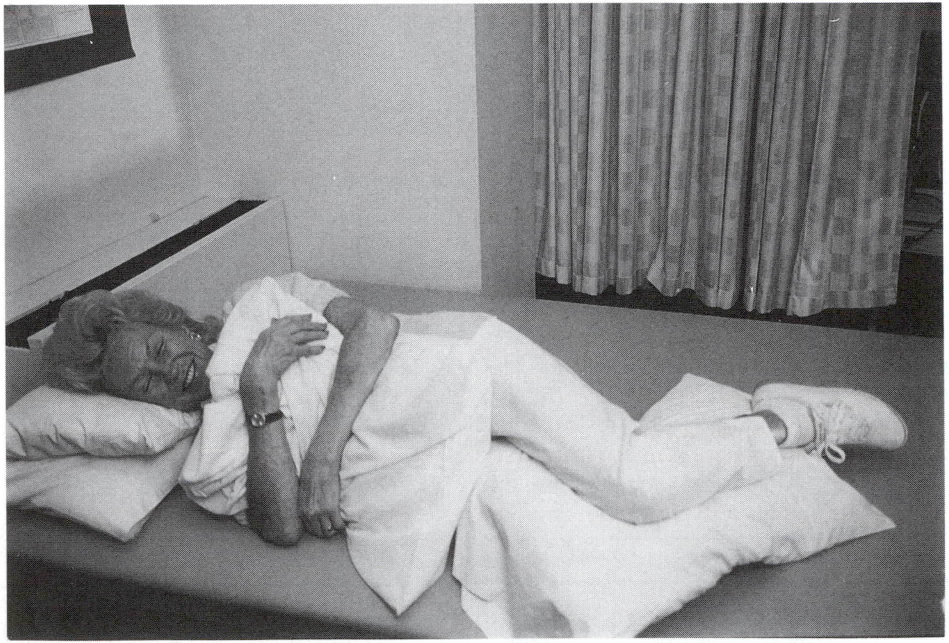

A. Sidelying position

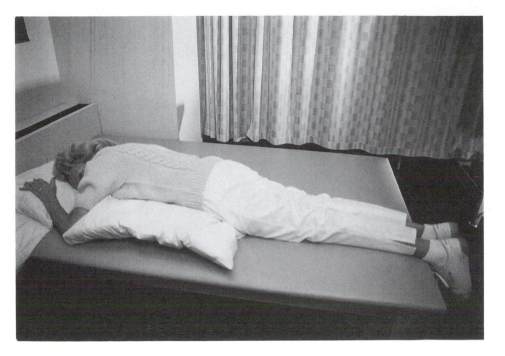

B. Prone position

continues

Figure 2-1 continued

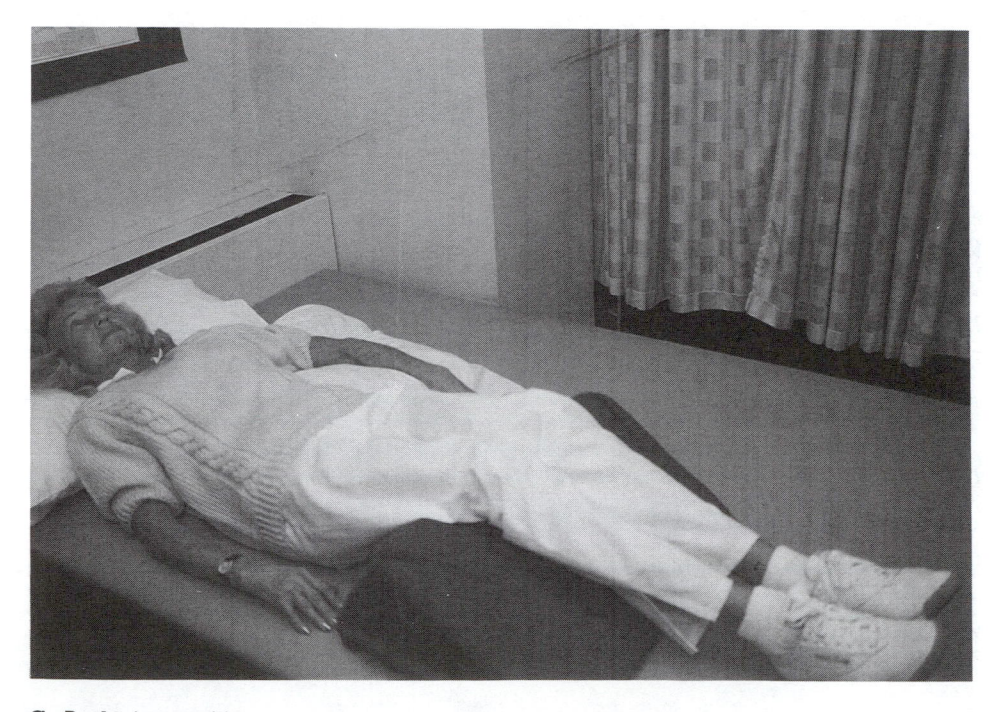

C. Backlying position

Figure 2-2 Progressive Position to Wean Patients Off the Supine Semi-Fowler Position

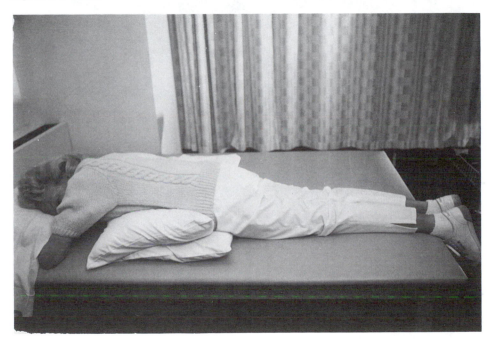

continues

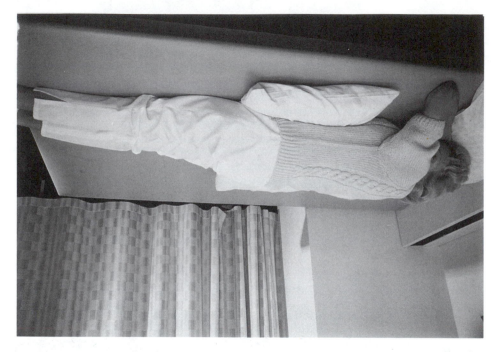

Figure 2-2 continued

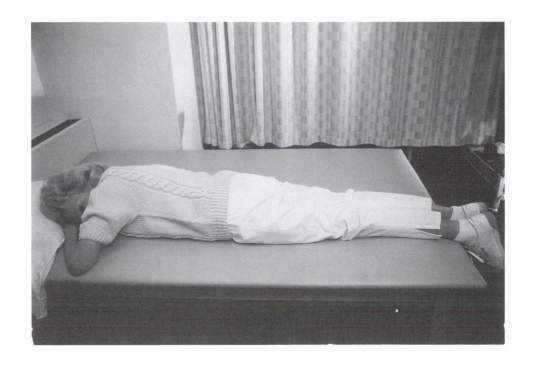

from the supine to the prone position. Some of them fall into general categories:

1. *upper extremity categories*
   - lift and reach below shoulder level
   - lift and reach above shoulder level
   - upper extremity push and reach
   - upper extremity push
2. *head and trunk categories*
   - right pelvis aligned with right shoulder girdle
   - right pelvis leads
   - relationship between pelvis and shoulder girdle changes
   - right shoulder girdle leads
3. *lower extremity categories*
   - bilateral lift
   - unilateral lift without a push
   - unilateral push
   - bilateral push.

The patterns listed first in each category are the ones most commonly used.

This information is valuable to rehabilitation spe-cialists because it supplies alternatives for evaluation and treatment. Rehabilitation specialists can identify a patient's movement pattern as described on this list and then a combination of therapeutic techniques to enhance the patient's rolling pattern or even to adapt the patient's pattern to one that the patient can tolerate more easily. Many elderly people tend to use the more rigid postures that keep the pelvis and the shoulders aligned. Rehabilitation specialists should identify this pattern and begin to facilitate the use of the pattern that is most comfortable for these individuals.

Many studies have shown that people can improve activity by visualizing body motions during the activity.[9–11] Before beginning treatment, the rehabilitation specialist may ask patients to warm up by picturing themselves rolling back and forth for five minutes. Patients should try to develop a clear image, "feel" the movement of their arms, legs, hips, and shoulders, and "sense" their contact with the sheets, covers, and air. The more detailed the visualization, the better. This kind of visualization prepares the patient for the activity.

In order to encourage motion in the bed activity,

the rehabilitation specialist should break the activity into its component parts. The hip slosh, for example, focuses on the hips. The person first does a pelvic tilt and then moves the hips from side to side, forward and backward, and around in circles. This helps patients begin to have a feeling of motion in their hip musculature. Bridges are also extremely important, and the patient should practice them almost every hour. Both upper and lower body bridges help the patient progress to the next stage of the mobility spectrum. Watching a demonstration of the exercises on a videotape while they are exercising may help patients increase their activity. Gentle rocking oscillations of various body parts to encourage even the smallest amount of motion can improve the patient's ability to turn over and move in bed.

Muscles particularly important for movement along the mobility spectrum are hip, knee, and ankle muscles. If classic progressive resistive exercises are not helpful, other stretching and strengthening techniques will be necessary. Electrical stimulation, quick stretch, overflow from other muscle groups (such as end of the range isometrics), and synergistic activities strengthen weak muscles. Exercises that require muscles to contract, relax, and contract again stretch and strengthen muscles at the same time.

In addition, gentle neck rotation while supine stimulates the cervical mechanoreceptors and establishes a stable base for the body proprioception that is required for standing.[12] Knee rocks (Figure 2–3) are helpful in loosening up the trunk. Encouraging the patient to work closer to the edge of the bed will help the patient overcome the fear of falling out of bed.

Once the appropriate muscles are being stretched and strengthened, and the patient is working hourly on bed activities (e.g., rocking, rolling, scooting, and visualizing), it is time to prepare for the next stage of the mobility spectrum: sitting. In order for the patient to do this in the bed mobility phase of treatment, the rehabilitation specialist should work with the patient on lateral flexing of the spine (often lost in stroke patients). It is also necessary to work on forward flexing of the trunk and the hips to prepare for vertical weight bearing in the next part of the mobility spectrum.

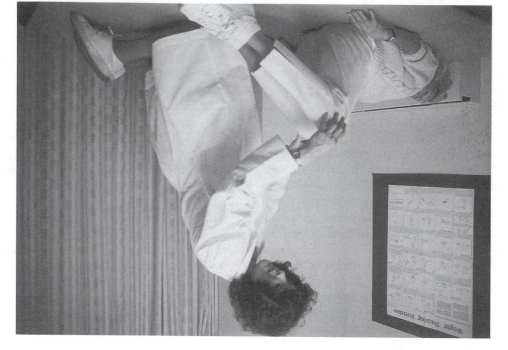

Figure 2-3 Knee Rocks

Bed Mobility

NOTES

1. N.L. Browse, *Pathology of Bed Rest* (Springfield, Ill.: Charles C Thomas, 1965).
2. M.A. Shepard, D. Parker, and N. DeClucque, "The Under-Reporting of Pressure Sores in Patients Transferred Between Hospital and Nursing Home," *Journal of the American Geriatric Society* 35 (1987): 159.
3. M. Miller and D. Elliott, "Errors and Omissions in Diagnostic Records on Admission of Patients to a Nursing Home," *Journal of the American Geriatric Society* 24 (1976): 108.
4. D. Gould, "Pressure Sore Prevention and Treatment," *Journal of Advances in Neurosurgery* 11 (1986): 389.
5. R. Lincoln et al., "Use of the Norton Pressure Sore Risk Assessment Scoring System with Elderly Patients in Acute Care," *Journal of Enterostom Therapy* 13 (1986): 13.
6. Ibid.
7. B. J. Dwyer, T. Snow, and E. McConnell, *Focus on Geriatric Care and Rehabilitation* 1, no. 3 (1987):
8. R.R. Richter, "Rolling from Supine to Prone." (Poster presentation at Washington University, St. Louis, Missouri, 1987).
9. J.V. Clark, "Effect of Mental Practice on the Development of a Certain Motor Skill," *Research Quarterly* 31 (1960): 560.
10. W.E. Twining, "Mental Practice and Physical Practice in Learning a Motor Skill," *Research Quarterly* 20 (1949): 434–35.
11. H. Wickman and P. Lizotte, "Effects of Mental Practice and Focus of Control on Performance of Dart Throwing," *Perceptual Motor Skills* 56 (1983): 807.
12. B. Wyke, "Cervical Articular Contributions to Posture and Gait: Their Relation to Senile Disequilibrium," *Age and Aging* 8 (1979): 251.

Sitting

III

Sitting is a key component of independence. This stage of the mobility spectrum can cause significant stress in the patient who has experienced cardiovascular deconditioning, and a patient who cannot sit without cardiovascular compromise obviously will never be able to stand, transfer, or ambulate.

CONDITIONING THE SITTER

In any program to rehabilitate a person with mobility problems, specific attention must be given to the patient's sitting tolerance. Essentially, the rehabilitation specialist conditions patients for sitting by having them sit for increasingly longer periods of time (Table 3–1). The patient can remain sitting as long as the heart rate remains below 100 beats per minute. If the heart rate rises above 100 beats per minute, the patient must lie down. Therefore, if a patient sits up for 5 minutes in the morning and his or her heart rate goes over 100 beats per minute, the patient may be allowed to sit up initially for 6 minutes in the afternoon with the heart rate monitored every 2 minutes. This procedure is repeated at successive sessions until the patient can tolerate sitting for 15 minutes.[1] Older patients should not be pushed too hard because this can cause too much stress on the cardiovascular system. This overload in a deconditioned patient is usually recognized as extreme fatigue later in the day.

Before beginning treatment, the rehabilitation specialist should know the patient's cardiovascular progression, (i.e., resting heart rate and normal increases of heart rate). For example, if a patient's heart rate is 60 beats per minute at rest, it should not rise above 85 beats per minute when the patient begins to sit; if the heart rate is 90 beats per minute at rest, it should not go over 120 beats per minute. When through sitting, the patient's heart

Table 3-1 Sitting Tolerance Schedule

Day	Time of Day	Activity
1	9 AM or 10 AM	Patient sits in chair or wheelchair for 15 minutes
	1 PM or 2 PM	Same activity for 30 minutes
	5 PM or 6 PM	Same activity for 45 minutes
2	9 AM or 10 AM	Patient sits in chair or wheelchair for 1 hour
	1 PM or 2 PM	Same activity for 1 hour 15 minutes
	5 PM or 6 PM	Same activity for 1 hour 30 minutes
3	9 AM or 10 AM	Patient sits in chair or wheelchair for 2 hours
	1 PM or 2 PM	Same activity for 2 hours 15 minutes
	5 PM or 6 PM	Same activity for 2 hours 30 minutes
4	9 AM or 10 AM	Patient sits in chair or wheelchair for 3 hours
	1 PM or 2 PM	Same activity for 3 hours 15 minutes
	5 PM or 6 PM	Same activity for 3 hours 30 minutes

Source: Reprinted from *Basic Rehabilitation Techniques: A Self-Instructional Guide,* 3rd ed., by R.D. Sine et al., p. 76, Aspen Publishers, Inc., © 1988.

rate should be in the range of 60 to 90 beats per minute.

The rehabilitation specialist should monitor patients' heart rate before they sit, while they sit, and when they have finished sitting. When patients are sitting, the rehabilitation specialist should watch for sudden changes in the speed, rate, and rhythm of the heart. In addition, the specialist should be on the alert for signs of cardiac problems, such as shortness of breath, pain in the chest, skin discoloration, nausea, dizziness, or sweating.

POSITIONING

The rehabilitation specialist should stress proper positioning for sitting (Figure 3–1). Positioning is important for all patients, as it helps to establish good muscle tone. When the patient is resting, the weight should be back and supported. When the sitting patient is active, the weight should be forward, communicating pressure and movement to the lower extremities in anticipation of weight bearing.

SITTING ACTIVITIES

Sitting activities can be divided into activities that:

- encourage body awareness
- prevent excessive pressure
- prepare for transfers
- improve cardiovascular status
- increase strength and range of motion.

Exercises to encourage body awareness can be accomplished through visualization. In visualization techniques, sitting patients simply think of how they are sitting in the chair and how they could improve this position. Exhibit 3–1 gives visualization suggestions. The use of small sitting movements can encourage awareness and prepare the sitter for standing.

An exercise to prevent excessive pressure is to have the patient shift his or her weight side to the side, lift off the seat, lean forward and backward,

Figure 3-1 Proper Positioning for Sitting

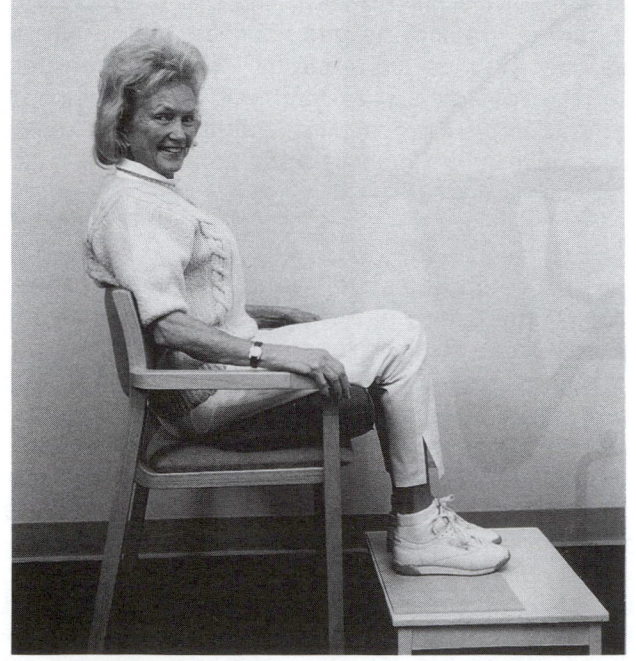

A. Resting sitting

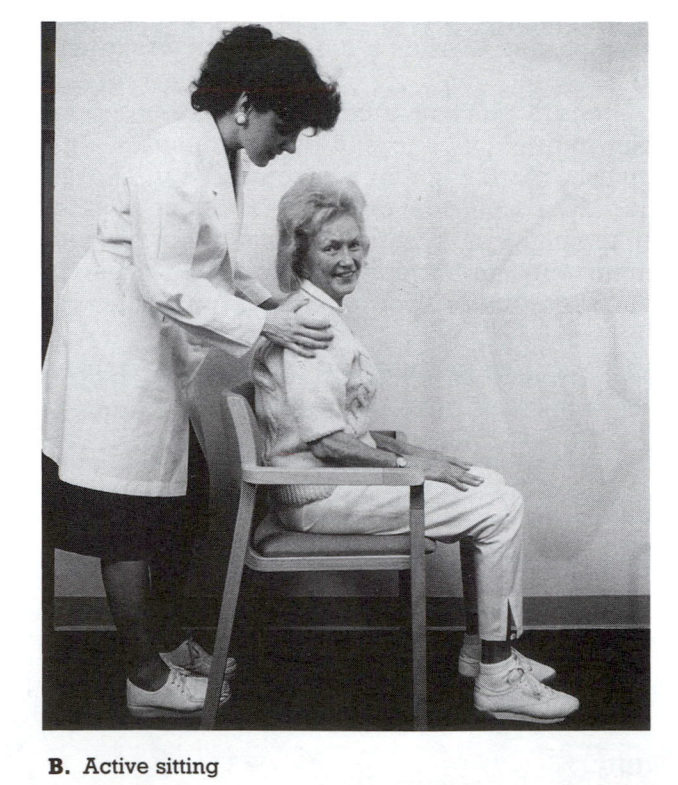

B. Active sitting

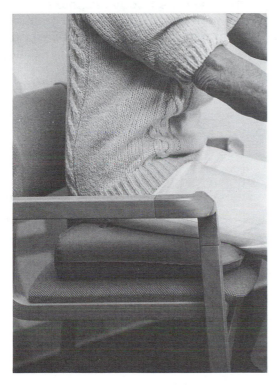

C. Wedge to enhance active sitting

Exhibit 3-1 Sitting Visualization

> Sit in your chair and feel where your sitting bones
>   touch the seat. Is one lighter than the other?
> Can you feel your thighs touching the chair?
> Is one thigh touching more of the chair? Which one?
>   How much more? On what part of the thigh?
> Now, gently slide one knee forward without lifting
>   your leg or moving your shoulders. Now slide
>   that knee back and the other knee forward.
> Feel which leg moves more easily.
> Feel where you are loose and where you are tight.

and scoot forward and backward at 20-minute intervals throughout the day.

Any additional movement improves a patient's cardiovascular status. A note of caution, however, is that upper body motions increase blood pressure more than lower body activities and therefore are recommended when patients can be monitored for an increase in blood pressure.[2] Leg motion exercises are useful in improving cardiovascular status, as are wheelchair exercises performed along with a videotaped exercise program. (See

Chapter 10.) Again, it is essential to monitor heart rate and blood pressure.[3]

Sitting activities that prepare the older person for transferring include:

- applying weight bearing pressure on lower extremities
- improving cardiovascular status
- visualizing the transfer
- increasing strength and range of motion in the lower extremities, the hips, and the upper extremities

Four strengthening and range of motion exercises are:

1. *Quadricep strengthening:* Extend the knee and hold for 10 seconds; do not hold breath; count aloud.
2. *Hip strengthening:* Lift the hips in the air and hold for 5 seconds (hip lifts); count aloud.
3. *Forward movement of the trunk on the hips*
   - Gently lean forward five times.
   - Gently lean forward and touch the knees; progress to touching calves and ankles.
4. *Seat mobility*
   - Scoot in the seat forward, backward, and from side to side.
   - Push up.
   - Rock forward and backward.

Exercises to increase strength are similar to those used to prepare for transfer (e.g., exercises to strengthen the quadriceps and the hips), but progressively greater weights are added. For motion, some gentle activities to loosen up the collagen and the joints can be helpful. For example, the Coke bottle roll, in which the patient gently rocks the foot forward and backward over a Coke bottle, helps keep the collagen loose in the hip and the knee (Figure 3–2).

SITTING BALANCE

Rather than push the patient around to train balance, the rehabilitation specialist should try a more normalized approach.[4] The patient's balance can

Figure 3-2 Coke Bottle Roll

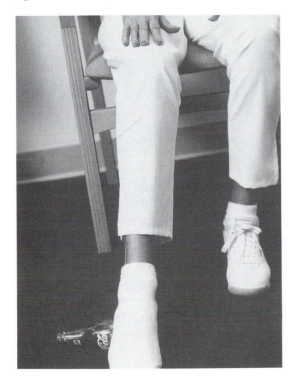

be assessed and treated at the same time if the rehabilitation specialist asks the patient to perform progressively more difficult sitting tasks:

1. Sit and look straight ahead.
2. Look at the ceiling.
3. Look to the right and to the left.
4. Look behind.
5. Reach for the
   - thigh
   - knee
   - calf
   - ankle.
6. Reach for the floor
   - in front
   - to each side.
7. Lean way back, way forward, and from side to side.

If the patient is free of pressure sores, can comfortably sit for one hour with good cardiovascular status, and has no balance problem, the sitting stage of the mobility spectrum will have been mastered. At this point, the rehabilitation specialist begins to work on activities that improve the range of motion, increase strength, and facilitate movement of the hip and the trunk in order to prepare the patient for the next phase of the mobility spectrum: transfers.

NOTES

1. R. Sine, *Basic Rehabilitation Techniques* (Rockville, Md.: Aspen Publishing, Inc., 1983).

2. C.B. Lewis, "Effects of Aging on the Cardiovascular System," *Clinical Management* 4, no. 4 (1984): 29–32.
3. Ibid.
4. J.H. Carr and R. Shephard, *A Motor Re-Learning Programme for Stroke,* 2nd ed. (Rockville, Md.: Aspen Publishers, Inc., 1987).

Transfers

IV

In a study to identify the factors that are most strongly correlated with admission to a nursing home, Keene and Anderson[1] found that a lack of cognitive ability, loss of control of the bowel and bladder, and the inability to transfer independently were the most frequent reasons for institutionalization. Therefore, people who are independent in transfers may be able to stay in their homes longer.

TRANSFER COMPONENTS

Unlike Richter,[2] who found variations in the way that people roll from the supine to the prone position, Nuzik et al.[3] found a good deal of similarity in the way that people transfer or get up and move from sitting to standing. Therefore, generalizations can be made about the complicated process of transfers.

Nuzik et al.[4] divided sit-to-stand transfers into two phases: the flexion phase and the extension phase. In the flexion phase, which is the first 35 percent of the activity, the person goes into neck and trunk flexion. In the remaining 65 percent of the sit-to-stand activity, the neck and trunk go into extension. The pelvis, which is initially posterior, rotates anteriorly. The hip is in flexion for the first 40 percent of the activity and goes into extension for the last 60 percent of the activity. The knees go into extension throughout the activity. The trunk moves vertically after 45 percent of the movement has taken place. The real key is that after 35 percent of the activity, the person begins to lift the hips off the seat. At that point, everything goes into extension. The hip lifting highlights the importance of hip extension in a patient's movement from sitting to standing.

TRANSFER EVALUATION

For evaluation, the rehabilitation specialist should examine the components of the transfer activity:

- What does the patient do when going from flexion into extension?
- Does the patient extend the head?
- Does the patient move the trunk?
- Do the hips flex for the first 40 percent of the activity or do they extend?

It is necessary to recognize that the patient must get the body over the hip area in order to have enough leverage to bring the body weight up. Although it is possible to stand up without flexing the trunk or the head, it is neither efficient nor easy.

A transfer evaluation form, such as that shown in Exhibit 4-1, may be extremely helpful to the rehabilitation specialist. In the section of the form on cardiopulmonary status, the rehabilitation specialist records the patient's resting heart rate and blood pressure and the end-of-session heart rate and blood pressure to ensure that the activities fall within the patient's cardiopulmonary limitations. In addition, the heart rate and the blood pressure are recorded when the patient stands to identify any orthostatic hypotension. The rehabilitation specialist should also note whether the patient uses the accessory, the sternocleidomastoid, or the scalenes muscles in breathing. The time required to complete the sit-to-stand activity should be recorded. The average time for this activity is 1.8 seconds.[5] A realistic short-term goal can be to shorten the length of time because the need for an unreasonable amount of time to go through the transfer process may limit the availability of standby assistance and, thus, hinder independence.

In the section on neuromusculoskeletal status, the rehabilitation specialist should note the muscle tone, strength, and flexibility and the need for assistance. It is particularly important to determine (1) whether the patient has enough hip strength or knee strength to stand, and (2) whether the patient is flexible enough in the hips and the knees to stand. In the section on sensory environment status,

Exhibit 4-1 Transfer Evaluation Form

Name _____

Date _____

Cardiopulmonary Status

    RHR _____   EHR _____

    RBP _____   EBP _____

    Sit-to-Stand HR _____   BP _____

    Sit-to-Stand Time _____

Neuromusculoskeletal Status

    Tone _____

    Strength _____

    Flexibility _____

Psychosocial Status

    Personal _____

    Support System _____

continues

Exhibit 4-1 continued

Transfer Position

	Initial	Middle	Ending
Head			
Neck			
Trunk			
Hips			
Pelvis			
Knees			
Feet			

Note: RHR, resting heart rate; *EHR,* end-of-session heart rate; *RBP,* resting blood pressure; *EBP,* end-of-session blood pressure; *HR,* heart rate; *BP,* blood pressure.

the rehabilitation specialist should note any fear, depression, or history of problems with transfer-ring. Is there a special reason the patient wants to transfer? What is the patient's support system? Who is there to help the patient at home? Are they not helpful enough or too helpful?

Finally, in the section of the form on transfer po-sition, the rehabilitation specialist should note the position of the various body parts. Notations for normal (N) or within normal limits (WNL) can be used as well as goniometric measures. Thus, if a person flexes the hips only 95 degrees initially and it is necessary to flex them 120 degrees, the short-term goal can be to achieve that additional 25 de-grees of flexion. It is essential, however, to avoid excessive spinal flexion when the patient is stand-ing so as to prevent pressure that may cause an osteoporotic compression fracture.

TRANSFER TECHNIQUES

In order to treat difficiencies in the transfer process, the rehabilitation specialist should begin working on activities that will facilitate the patient's ability to perform the component motions. For example, initial activities may include:

- leaning the body weight forward
- putting weight forward on the hip
- bending the head forward then extending
- extending the knee while extending the trunk

Some techniques that focus on middle to ending motions are:

- hip lifts off the chair
- rocking trunk from flexion to extension
- knee extension exercises
- standing hip extensions
- hip thrusts combined with head extensions

It is important to teach both flexion and extension. The rehabilitation specialist should analyze the task to determine where the hips work, where the knees work, and how they work, so that treatment focuses on the appropriate phase of the activity (Table 4-1).

Working on hip movement generally improves the anterior movement of the pelvis, as well as trunk and knee flexion. Bobath[6] recommended having patients slide their hands along a chair in front of them to encourage flexion of the trunk for the first 30 to 40 percent of a stand (Figure 4-1). In addition, having a chair in front of them makes fearful patients more confident. If a patient is not motivated to transfer, it is sometimes helpful to place a colorful and attractive print or blanket on the chair to which the patient is transferring. Putting a familiar blanket on the transfer object can also motivate movement.

An important part of attaining and maintaining the upright position is input from the autonomic nervous system. Increased activity of the sympathetic nervous system interferes with the patient's

Table 4-1 Mean Angular Positions Computed at Five-Percent Intervals of the Sit-to-Stand Movement Pattern (in Degrees)

Interval	Movement Pattern (%)	Ankle[a]		Knee[a]		Hip[a]		Pelvis[b]		Trunk[b]		Neck[b]		Frankfort[b] Plane	
		$\overline{X}$	s	$\overline{X}$	s	$\overline{X}$	s	$\overline{X}$	s	$\overline{X}$	s	$\overline{X}$	s	$\overline{X}$	s
Start	0	105.75	6.59	94.61	5.83	135.25	11.55	116.25	10.51	79.78	6.46	62.63	7.94	−2.10	11.94
1	5	105.56	6.72	94.53	5.79	134.57	11.65	115.62	10.56	79.15	6.52	61.93	7.94	−2.61	11.78
2	10	105.23	6.79	94.56	5.81	133.24	11.62	114.28	10.48	77.66	6.55	60.81	8.06	−3.25	11.81
3	15	104.75	6.75	94.57	5.84	130.87	11.53	111.79	10.31	74.83	6.62	59.14	8.28	−4.03	11.95
4	20	104.10	6.63	94.68	5.89	126.94	11.40	107.53	10.14	70.39	6.80	57.09	8.65	−4.80	12.30
5	25	103.26	6.51	95.06	5.94	121.54	11.18	101.33	9.92	64.77	7.21	55.19	9.33	−5.51	12.82
6	30	102.21	6.42	96.02	5.96	115.70	10.80	93.80	9.46	58.62	7.82	53.93	10.37	−5.84	13.59
7	35	101.03	6.35	97.89	5.99	111.60	10.28	86.75	8.59	53.20	8.77	53.40	11.54	−5.71	14.36
8	40	99.93	6.26	101.08	6.20	110.88	10.28	81.65	7.95	49.52	9.90	53.47	12.47	−5.27	14.95
9	45	99.31	6.13	105.90	6.61	113.73	10.64	78.88	7.52	48.22	11.00	54.18	12.88	−4.52	15.09
10	50	99.44	5.98	112.47	7.26	119.39	11.21	77.89	7.33	49.40	11.75	55.64	12.68	−3.38	14.74
11	55	100.28	5.83	120.32	7.75	126.81	11.46	78.11	7.16	52.66	11.90	57.76	11.98	−1.87	13.92
12	60	101.68	5.79	129.07	8.35	135.35	11.41	79.13	6.90	57.55	11.53	60.36	10.99	−0.13	12.87
13	65	103.44	5.78	138.21	8.94	144.33	10.97	80.62	6.53	63.44	10.60	62.98	9.86	1.49	11.79
14	70	105.30	5.79	147.20	9.15	153.19	10.04	82.30	6.12	69.72	9.22	65.27	8.91	2.73	10.95
15	75	107.19	5.63	155.75	9.01	161.49	9.25	83.95	5.84	75.90	7.61	66.94	8.28	3.36	10.39
16	80	108.87	5.31	163.11	8.08	168.60	8.24	85.41	5.61	81.33	6.06	68.08	7.79	3.55	9.91
17	85	110.21	4.94	169.06	6.86	174.32	7.54	86.59	5.45	85.65	4.95	68.88	7.45	3.59	9.56
18	90	111.12	4.67	173.46	5.78	178.68	7.01	87.53	5.30	88.86	4.25	69.54	7.22	3.71	9.43
19	95	111.59	4.51	176.22	5.17	181.56	6.77	88.17	5.18	91.00	3.88	70.09	7.15	3.78	9.31
20	100	111.74	4.45	177.86	4.98	183.40	6.74	88.58	5.13	92.49	3.65	70.06	7.21	3.67	9.28

[a] Values define the angular measurements between body segments as delineated by data points.
[b] Angular measurements reflect the relationship of the body segment to the positive x axis.

Source: Reprinted from ''Sit-to-Stand Movement Pattern: A Kinematic Study'' by S. Nuzik et al. in *Physical Therapy,* Vol. 66, No. 11, p. 1709, with permission of American Physical Therapy Association, © 1986.

Figure 4-1 Facilitating Flexion in Sit-To-Stand Movements

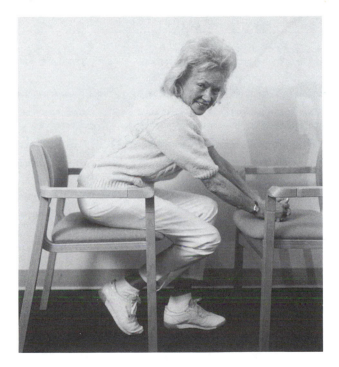

ability to perform low-energy phasic movements (e.g., transferring) or to hold low-energy tonic patterns (e.g., standing). Some patients tend to go into the extensor pattern and are unable to go into flexion. Such patients, particularly older patients, may be functioning in the sympathetic mode (Table 4-2)[7]; if so, they may have a rapid or increased pulse, dilated pupils, and an extensor tone. In order to overcome the extension pattern, the rehabilitation specialist must first help the patient function in a parasympathetic mode. In other words, it is necessary to help the patient relax so that the muscle tone can be more normal.

Rood[8] introduced several techniques to stimulate the parasympathetic system and decrease extension tones: gentle thoracic stroking; midline touch; or soft, slow talking for only 30 seconds (Figure 4-2); they encourage the patient to relax.[9] Deep diaphragmatic breathing can also be helpful, as it stimulates the vagus nerve, which causes parasympathetic firing. In one such activity, the rehabilitation specialist ensures that the patient is comfortably seated and then instructs the patient:

Table 4-2 Characteristics of the Autonomic Nervous System

	Sympathetic Mode	*Parasympathetic Mode*
Lung (respiration)	Shallow, rapid, and/or irregular breathing pattern	Slow, rhythmical diaphragmatic breathing pattern
Pulse	Rapid or increased	Slower or decreased from initial level
Eye		
Pupils	Dilated	Constricted
Eyelid	Elevated	
Sweating	Mild to profuse, usually on the hands or feet; chest and back	Dry skin, especially palms and soles of feet
Peripheral circulation	Decreased; distal extremities feel cold and clammy	Normal; distal extremities feel warm and dry
Digestive system	Decreased secretion of digestive enzymes	Increased secretion of digestive enzymes
Thymus and spleen (immune system)	Immune responsiveness regulated through transmitter influences on lymphocytes; tendency to develop infection	
Spontaneous movement	Frequent extraneous movement of extremities; tendency toward hyperkinetic	Relaxed, infrequent purposeless motion
Response to phasic touch	Away-from response: pulling away from touch in an exaggerated phasic movement pattern, high-energy phasic response	Low energy phasic response

Figure 4-2 Techniques to Decrease Extension Tone

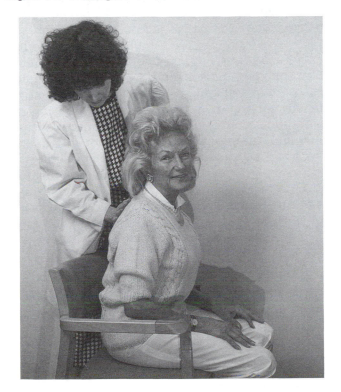

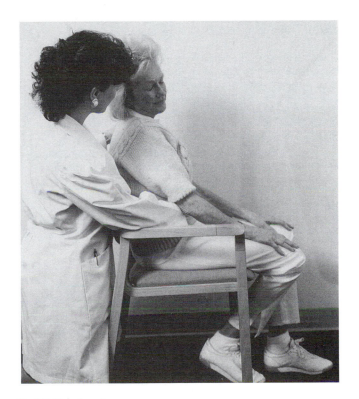

A. Gentle thoracic stroking done slowly for 30 seconds

B. Midline touch

- to breathe in and out diaphragmatically
- to say "my body is calm" and visualize on each inhalation
- to say "my body is quiet" and visualize on each exhalation
- to repeat this procedure five times

This activity generally has a calming effect and can be repeated 10 times throughout the day as a stress management technique.[10]

Adams[11] suggested that patients be placed in a prone position in order to move them from an extensor position into a more flexed position before treatment begins. According to Adams, patients should lie prone for 15 to 20 minutes. If the patient cannot tolerate the prone position, flexing the patient's head for as long as the patient can tolerate is helpful.

Once relaxed, the patient can try to transfer. The rehabilitation specialist should work with the older patient to encourage the proper sit-to-stand position and to strengthen the muscles needed for the activity. It is also necessary to consider the neuro-logical system in helping the patient to do the transfer activity properly. This encourages proper progressive standing.

NOTES

1. J.S. Keene and C.A. Anderson, "Hip Fractures in the Elderly: Discharge Predictions with a Functional Rating Scale," *Journal of the American Medical Association* 248 (1982): 564.
2. R.R. Richter, "Rolling from Supine to Prone." (Poster presentation at the American Physical Therapy Association Annual Meeting, San Antonio, Texas, June 1987).
3. S. Nuzik et al., "Sit-to-Stand Movement Pattern," *Physical Therapy* 66, no. 11 (1986): 1540–1541.
4. Ibid.
5. Ibid.
6. B. Bobath, "The Bobath Approach: Assessment and Treatment Planning." Videotape, University of Maryland, School of Physical Therapy, 1981, funded by the Administration on Aging.
7. C. Burnett, "Neurological Implications in Aging." (Continuing Education Course, Presented to the District of Columbia Physical Therapy Association, 1986).
8. M. Rood, Lecture Notes from "Therapeutic Exercise Techniques," Ohio State University, 1975.
9. Ibid.

10. G. Everly and D. Gerdano, *Controlling Stress and Tension: A Holistic Approach* (Englewood Cliffs, N.J.: Prentice-Hall, 1979).
11. G. Adams, *Essentials of Geriatric Medicine* (New York: Oxford University Press, 1977).

Standing Posture V

Many people spend a great deal of time standing, either in a static position or in a dynamic, balanced, action-ready position. For example, a grocery store cashier spends hours a day standing and moving from the standing position. This person is potentially vulnerable to many musculoskeletal problems, such as low back pain, knee pain, sore feet, and generalized stiffness.

STATIC STANDING POSTURE

"Good," or balanced, static posture is a matter of alignment. The head should be straight over the shoulders, the hips, the knees, and the ankles (Figure 5-1). As people age, however, they begin to have a more forward head, a greater rounding of the shoulders, and either flattening or hollowing of the lumbar spine, as well as an increase in hip and knee flexion (Figure 5-2).[1] These changes can

cause an older person to have significant problems with standing and walking.

Evaluation of Static Standing Posture

The rehabilitation specialist can evaluate static standing posture with a plumbline (see Figure 5-1). The patient stands sideways to the plumbline with the anchor point just medial to and slightly in front of the lateral malleolus. The rehabilitation specialist notes and ranks any postural deviations on a scale from 0 to 10, as shown at the top column of each for every body part, beginning with the ear, the shoulder, the hip, the knee, and the ankle. The patient then turns so that the rehabilitation specialist has a full front or back view, with the plumbline directly bisecting the patient's body. At this point, the rehabilitation specialist evaluates the symmetry of the body position.

Figure 5-1 Alignment of Good Posture

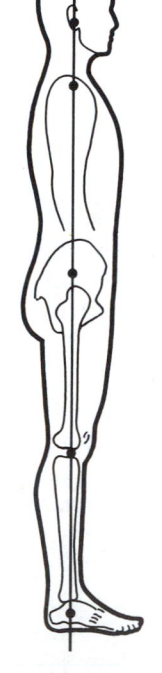

A plumbline bisects the

middle of the ear; goes through

the acromion process,

the greater trochanter, and

a point just behind the patella; to

a point just anterior to the lateral malleolus

Figure 5-2 Posture Changes with Age

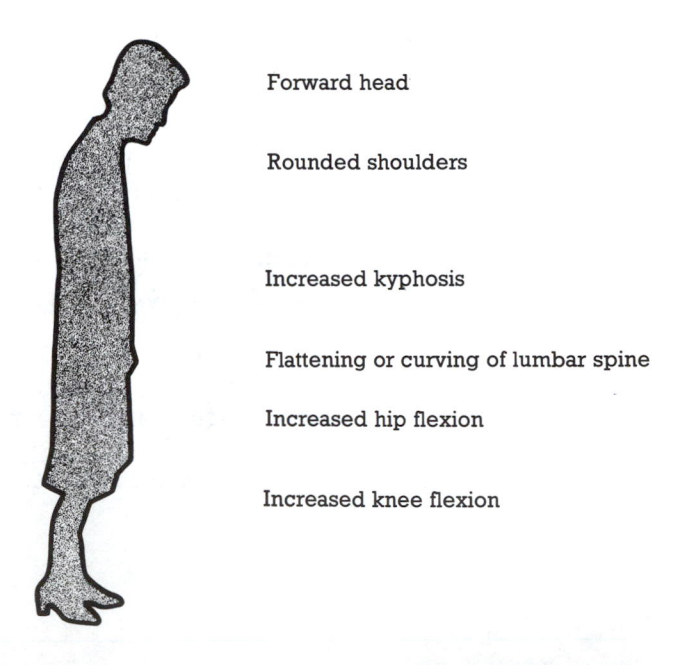

Forward head

Rounded shoulders

Increased kyphosis

Flattening or curving of lumbar spine

Increased hip flexion

Increased knee flexion

A posture grid can be used in conjunction with the plumbline to assess body position by even smaller segments, or the Reedco posture evaluation tool can be used (Figure 5-3). The rehabilitation specialist can use this tool to rate posture at the various body parts (e.g. head, neck, shoulder, hip, and ankle) on a scale of 0 to 10. For example, a patient whose head is very slightly deviated to the left may receive an 8 rating on head position. Two modifications may be added to the Reedco evaluation sheet:

1. Flat backs can be assessed as part of the lower back category, with a score of 5 (fair) indicating a slightly flat back and a score of 0 (poor) indicating a markedly flat back.
2. An assessment of knee, hip, and ankle position from the lateral view can be added at the bottom of the page. The best way to assess these positions is with a goniometer (e.g., hip flexion, 20 degree; knee flexion, 15 degree; ankle dorsiflexion, 5 degree).

Such tools permit a specific evaluation of a patient's posture and a specific ranking grade. This information can be used to determine the way in which the patient's posture affects his or her mobility as well as comfort for daily activities.

Treatment of Problems with Static Standing Posture

Once a patient's posture has been evaluated, the rehabilitation specialist can design a program to improve posture. Such a program should include several types of:

- chin tucks to move a forward head back (Figure 5-4)
- shoulder rolls, shoulder shrugs, or scapular retraction to improve rounded shoulders (Figure 5-5)
- extension exercises to increase lumbar lordosis (Figure 5-6)
- pelvic tilts to flatten the lumbar spine
- lower body extension exercises to improve hip and knee extension (Figure 5-7)

Figure 5-3 Posture Evaluation Score Sheet

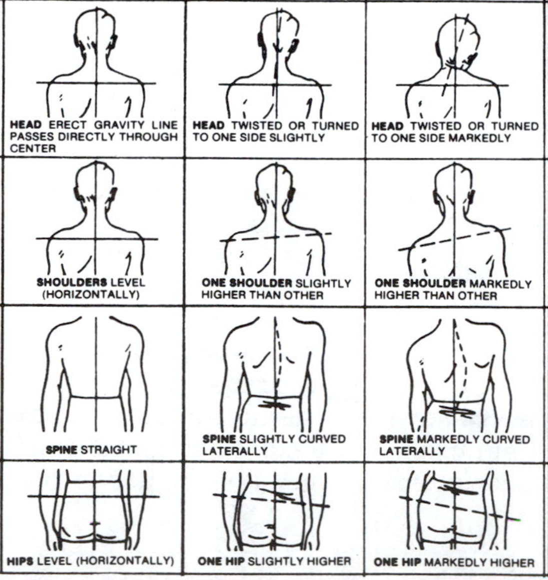

POSTURE SCORE SHEET	Name _____			SCORING DATES			
	GOOD - 10	FAIR - 5	POOR - 0				
HEAD LEFT RIGHT	HEAD ERECT GRAVITY LINE PASSES DIRECTLY THROUGH CENTER	HEAD TWISTED OR TURNED TO ONE SIDE SLIGHTLY	HEAD TWISTED OR TURNED TO ONE SIDE MARKEDLY				
SHOULDERS LEFT RIGHT	SHOULDERS LEVEL (HORIZONTALLY)	ONE SHOULDER SLIGHTLY HIGHER THAN OTHER	ONE SHOULDER MARKEDLY HIGHER THAN OTHER				
SPINE LEFT RIGHT	SPINE STRAIGHT	SPINE SLIGHTLY CURVED LATERALLY	SPINE MARKEDLY CURVED LATERALLY				
HIPS LEFT RIGHT	HIPS LEVEL (HORIZONTALLY)	ONE HIP SLIGHTLY HIGHER	ONE HIP MARKEDLY HIGHER				

ANKLES	FEET POINTED STRAIGHT AHEAD	FEET POINTED OUT	FEET POINTED OUT MARKEDLY ANKLES SAG IN (PRONATION)				
NECK	NECK ERECT, CHIN IN, HEAD IN BALANCE DIRECTLY ABOVE SHOULDERS	NECK SLIGHTLY FORWARD, CHIN SLIGHTLY OUT	NECK MARKEDLY FORWARD, CHIN MARKEDLY OUT				
UPPER BACK	UPPER BACK NORMALLY ROUNDED	UPPER BACK SLIGHTLY MORE ROUNDED	UPPER BACK MARKEDLY ROUNDED				
TRUNK	TRUNK ERECT	TRUNK INCLINED TO REAR SLIGHTLY	TRUNK INCLINED TO REAR MARKEDLY				
ABDOMEN	ABDOMEN FLAT	ABDOMEN PROTRUDING	ABDOMEN PROTRUDING AND SAGGING				
LOWER BACK	LOWER BACK NORMALLY CURVED	LOWER BACK SLIGHTLY HOLLOW	LOWER BACK MARKEDLY HOLLOW				
ALL REPRODUCTION RIGHTS RESERVED © REEDCO "The Good Posture People" 51 NORTH FULTON ST. AUBURN, NY 13021 (315) 252-0020 COPYRIGHT 1974		**TOTAL SCORES**					

Figure 5-4 Chin Tucks

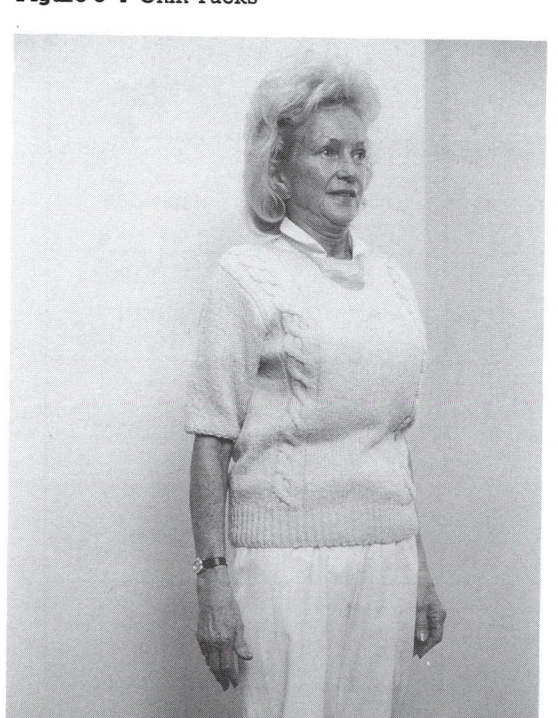

In addition, exercises to stretch hip flexors can be done gradually and in a variety of ways (Figure 5-8).

Posture improvement can be taught in a class setting by means of a lecture-demonstration-discussion format. Initially, there is a 10-minute lecture on good posture and modifications.[2] This is followed by a quick individual posture analysis and appropriate exercises. The final segment of the class is allotted to questions and answers on posture.[3]

When treating problems with static standing posture, the rehabilitation specialist must remember the following:

- Patients must be aware that postural improvement is likely to be slow.

- Posture correction requires frequent short bouts of exercise (e.g., two or three repetitions three to ten times a day).

- Feedback helps in posture correction. Patients should be encouraged to use mirrors and to help each other.

Figure 5-5 Exercises to Improve Rounded Shoulders

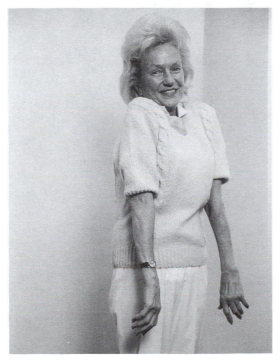

A. Shoulder Rolls

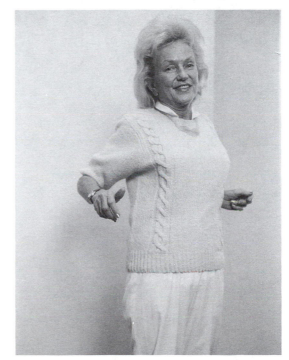

B. Shoulder Shrugs

55

continues

Figure 5-5 continued

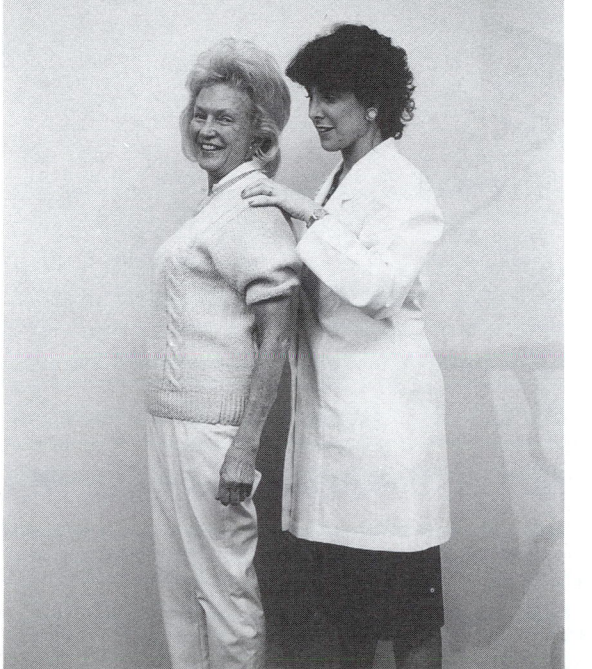

C. Scapular Retraction

Figure 5-6 Lumbar Extension Exercises

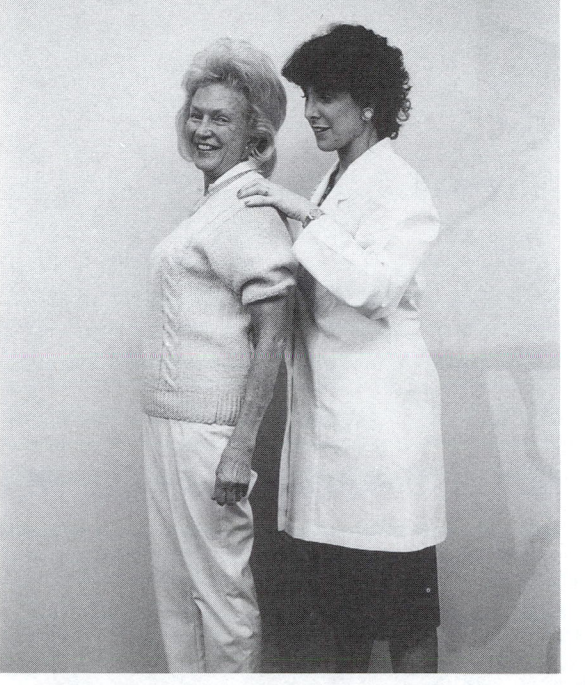

Figure 5-7 Lower Body Extension Exercises

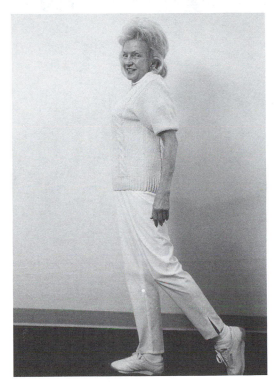

- If a person spends a great deal of time standing, the environment should be modified to alleviate musculoskeletal stress (see Figure 5-9).

DYNAMIC STANDING POSTURE

A much more elusive concept than static standing posture, dynamic standing posture involves a person's preparation for movement. Patients who can stand in a balanced, action-ready position are better able to use their body in performing activities. Therefore, the rehabilitation specialist must keep in mind two general questions when evaluating and treating the dynamic standing posture of older persons:

1. Are the muscles balanced and comfortable in the static position?
2. Is the musculoskeletal system in the optimal position for the action the body is about to perform?

For example, when starting to walk, is the person initiating the movement from the hips (are the hips,

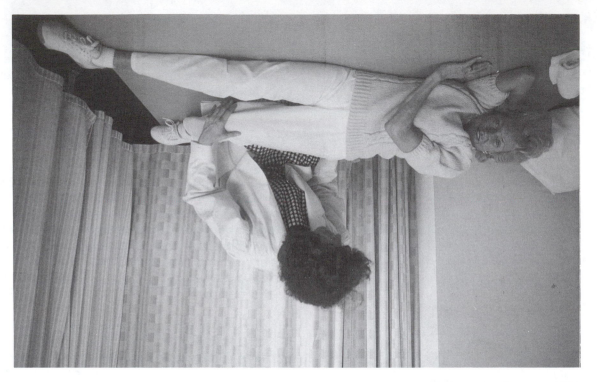

Figure 5-8 Hip Flexor Stretches

Standing Posture

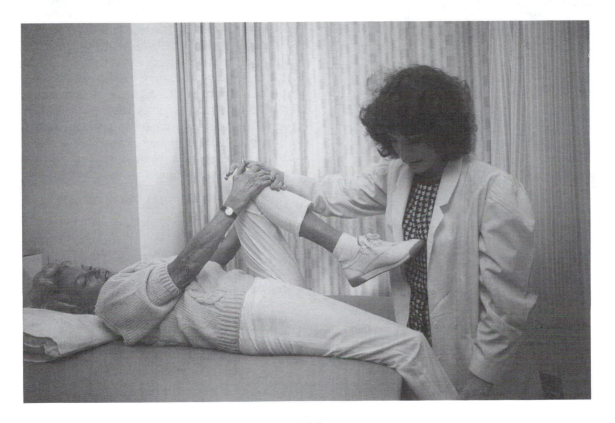

the trunk, and the head at a 30-degree angle, or is the person initiating the movement with the entire body (see Figure 5-10)? Because older persons may well have decreased energy reserves, movement that uses the body to encourage motion can improve their functioning. For example, a gentle leaning forward from the ankles when walking creates a forward momentum.

Evaluation of Dynamic Standing Posture

When assessing dynamic posture, the rehabilitation specialist should consider each activity in terms of body mechanics. For example, it is necessary to determine whether an older person who is working at the kitchen sink is using his or her body to help with the activity or is shifting weight when reaching and lifting. Thus, the evaluation of dynamic standing is simply assessing the patient's standing position as an activity is initiated. The evaluator looks at how this starting position helps or hinders the activity. The rehabilitation specialist should observe what the patient does while standing (e.g., meal preparation) and look for ways that the patient can facilitate the motions.

Figure 5-9 Modification of the Environment

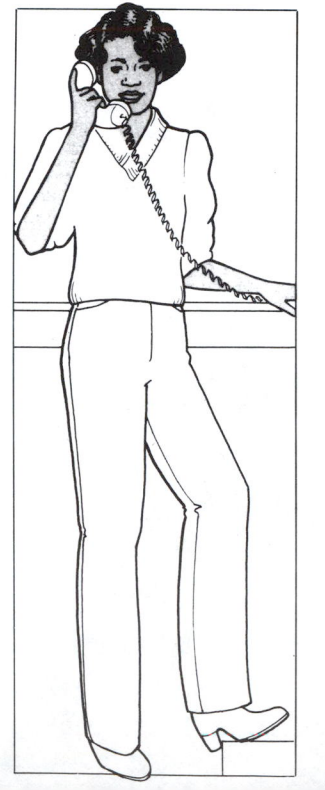

Placing one foot slightly higher than the other helps to relieve the back from the stress of standing for a long time.

Figure 5-10 Dynamic Standing: Starting to Walk
A. Inefficient Use of Movement

B. Good Use of Movement

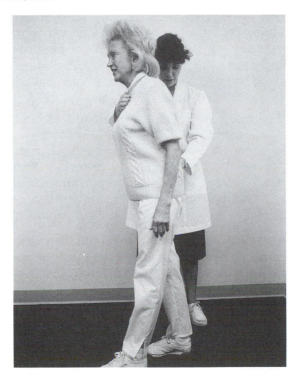

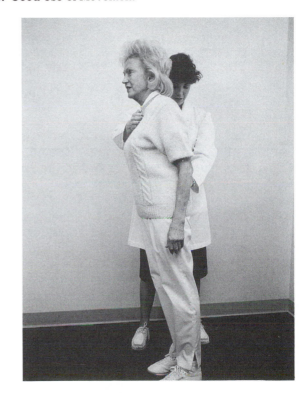

Treatment of Problems with Dynamic Standing Posture

The treatment for dysfunction or discomfort caused by problems with dynamic standing posture is to help the patient find better ways to move:

- A woman with a significant forward head has severe neck pain. Her pain gets worse when she stands and cooks but is relieved when she rests her head by sitting or lying down. Positional testing reveals that she feels much better with her head in a chin tuck position. A program of postural exercise and stretching will help this woman.

- A man with a severe forward head loses his balance when he begins to walk from a sitting or standing position. When he does a chin tuck, he puts his weight in a more centered position and does not lose his balance. Clearly, learning to stretch into a chin tuck and practicing a postural regime will help this man.

Unlike these two patients, some patients have made use of their postural deviations. For example, a patient with a forward head may find that the forward head position makes it easier to look through bifocals when walking with a walker. In this case, the postural deviation may actually help the patient see better and walk more safely. Therefore, changing posture in this patient may be inappropriate.

Rehabilitation specialists should apply the principles of body mechanics to the activities of daily living to break down tasks and, thus, to improve activity efficiency in older persons. Such task analyses and applications will set the stage for the next phase of the mobility spectrum: walking.

NOTES

1. C. Lewis, "Musculoskeletal Aspects of Aging," *Aging Health Care Challenge* (Philadelphia: F.A. Davis, 1984).
2. *Reedco Posture Score Sheet* (Auburn, N.Y.: Reedco Co., 1974).
3. C. Lewis and L. Campanelli, *Designing Rehabilitation Exercise Classes* (Rockville, Md.: Aspen Publishers, Inc., 1988).

Gait

VI

Gait is simply the loss and the recovery of balance. It is the body's way of using inertia to achieve efficient, effortless walking. Many of the gait problems of the elderly originate in their inability to maximize inertia and use gravity effectively.

BASIC TASKS IN WALKING

The three basic tasks in walking are:

1. weight acceptance
2. single limb support
3. limb advancement [1]

The first task involves great impact and requires control. As the swing leg is about to contact the ground, the hamstring and the quadricep muscles work together to slow the leg and steady it in preparation for weight acceptance. Because this is a vigorous and dynamic part of the gait cycle, the muscles involved must be strong. Unfortunately, studies indicate that the elderly have lost strength in the muscles needed for this activity.[2]

The four groups of muscles most active at the point of weight acceptance are (1) hip extensors, (2) hip abductors, (3) quadriceps, and (4) plantar flexors.[3] In "normal" older persons, quadricep strength is decreased by 28 percent and abductor strength by 38 percent.[4] If an older person experiences pain while walking, quadricep strength may be reduced by as much as 47 percent.[5] When these muscles are weak, various compensations occur. For example, the person may (1) decrease stride length, (2) lean forward from the hips to decrease flexion torque and lessen impact, and (3) decrease plantar flexion. Therefore, strengthening the four muscle groups involved may help improve the gait aspect of weight acceptance.

Single limb support requires strength in the hip abductors and in the limb so that the pelvis can be level and hold up the hip and the leg. If the abductors are weak, the trunk will shift to the weak side. This will help the person complete the phase of single limb support, but it may produce low back problems and an inefficient gait pattern. In addition, older persons spend 38 percent of the gait cycle in single limb support as opposed to 40 percent spent by normal young persons.[6]

Limb advancement requires not only flexibility and strength in the previously mentioned muscle groups but also plantar flexion. If the plantar flexors are weak, the stride length will decrease and a steppage gait may develop.

GAIT CHANGES IN THE ELDERLY

Problems in performing the basic tasks of walking may lead to gait changes in the elderly population:

- fewer automatic movements
- decreased speed and amplitude of automatic movements

- increased muscle activity in the gait cycle
- less accuracy and slower movement, especially in the hip
- decreased swing-to-stance ratio
- decreased vertical displacement
- broader stride width
- increased toe-floor clearance
- decrease heal-floor angle
- slower cadence
- decreased rotation of the hips and the shoulders
- more abnormalities in posture
- mild rigidity, particularly in proximal regions [7]

In addition to these changes, there is a 14 percent decrease in the speed of the ambulator[8] and a reduction in stride length. While stride length is generally 1.5 meters in young persons, it is 1.3 meters in normal elderly persons and 1.1 meters in elderly persons who have a pathological condition.[9]

The elderly experience an overall decrease in the range of motion that can affect gait. The general 5-degree decrease in the motion of the hips, the knees, and the ankles, for example, can alter the efficiency of the musculoskeletal system in walking.[10] Walters, Perry, and McDaniels[11] found that the strength of hip extensor muscles at 15-degree flexion is 41 percent greater than their strength when the hips are in full extension. Thus, a slight flexion of the hips may help a patient achieve a stronger extension in the gait cycle.

Finally, because of the noted gait changes, the actual task of walking may require more energy. The normal energy requirement for walking is 0.16 ml O_2/kg/min. In healthy older persons, it is 0.23 ml O_2/kg/min.[12] This is not a tremendous difference, but it is a difference that could be significant, especially in an older person who has a health problem.

EVALUATION OF GAIT

Careful evaluation of the components of gait and compensatory mechanisms is essential. The numerous techniques available for evaluating gait changes range from those that use sophisticated electronic equipment to subjective gait analysis. In subjective gait analysis, the rehabilitation specialist must be sure to consider the phase of gait (i.e., weight acceptance, single limb support, and limb advancement) as well as the components of gait and the body parts used:

1. heel strike
2. toe off
3. terminal extension of the knee
4. hip flexion and extension
5. trunk rotation
6. automatic movements

The rehabilitation specialist should note deficits and rate them separately on a 0 to 10 scale with 10 being normal gait characteristics and 0 being severely abnormal.

Objective gait analysis can be done through the use of Nelson's Functional Ambulation Profile (FAP) (Exhibit 6-1).[13] A quiet, flat area and a stop watch are required for the administration of the

Exhibit 6-1 Modified Functional Ambulation Profile

Patient: _____

STATIC WEIGHT-BEARING CAPACITY

Date							
Bilateral Time							
Left Unilateral Time							
Right Unilateral Time							

DYNAMIC (in place) WEIGHT TRANSFER RATE

Date							
Time to Complete 4 transfers (8 steps)							

BASIC AMBULATION EFFICIENCY

Date							
Through // bars Holding on time/steps							
Through // bars not holding on time/steps							
Twelve foot distance outside // bars time/steps							

COMMENTS

Content Addendum

Source: Reprinted from *Physical Therapy,* Vol. 54, p. 1061, with permission of American Physical Therapy Association, © 1974.

FAP. In the first section, static weight-bearing capacity, the rehabilitation specialist records the patient's ability to stand first on both legs (bilateral) for a maximum of 2 minutes, then on each leg (unilateral) for 30 seconds each. The patient then closes the eyes and repeats the task; the inability to balance on one leg with the eyes closed indicates that the patient used the eyes in the balance process.

The next section of the FAP, dynamic (in place) weight transfer rate, is used to record gait measures. The patient takes eight steps in place while the rehabilitation specialist times the ability.

In the final section, basic ambulation efficiency, the rehabilitation specialist records the time and the number of steps that the patient takes to walk through parallel bars or a measured distance. The bottom portion of this form is for comments, such as notes on deviations, endurance problems, or assistive devices.[14]

The FAP can be repeated in a week or a month for the objective measurement of the patient's improvement in gait training. The rehabilitation spe-

cialist must ensure the patient's safety while testing but should not provide physical support for balance. If physical assistance is necessary, the test should be modified and the same procedure repeated in subsequent FAP evaluations to ensure reliability.

TREATMENT STRATEGIES

Once the patient's gait has been thoroughly evaluated, the rehabilitation specialist can institute a regimen. Patients, particularly older patients, should be prepared or conditioned for gait training. The session should begin with warm-ups. Hip exercises, such as hip clocks (i.e., standing and making circles with the hips), are often good initial activities (Figure 6-1). It is also necessary to work on plantar flexion and dorsiflexion in conjunction with hip and lower extremity stretching and strengthening exercises (Figure 6-2).

Another good warm-up activity is to ask patients to visualize themselves walking down the hall. The patients should vividly imagine their successful

Figure 6-1 Warm-Up Exercises for Gait Training (Hip Slosh and Hip Clocks)

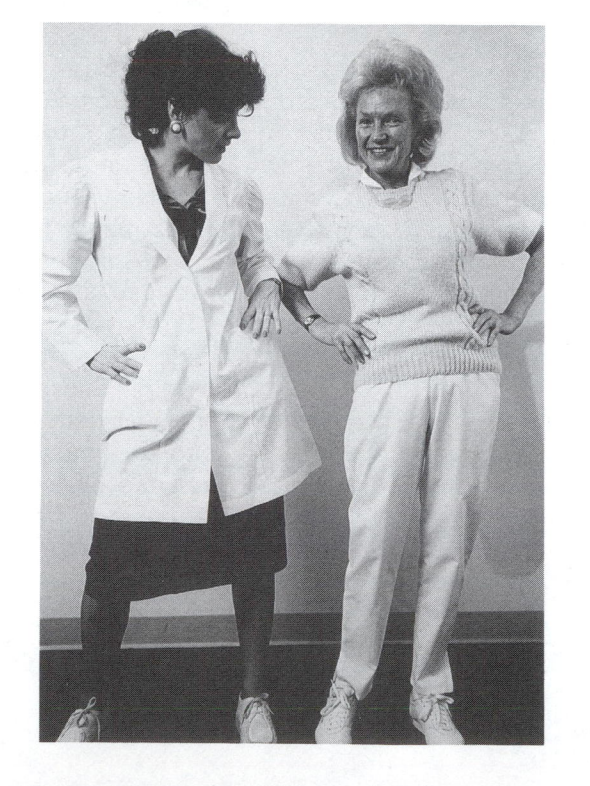 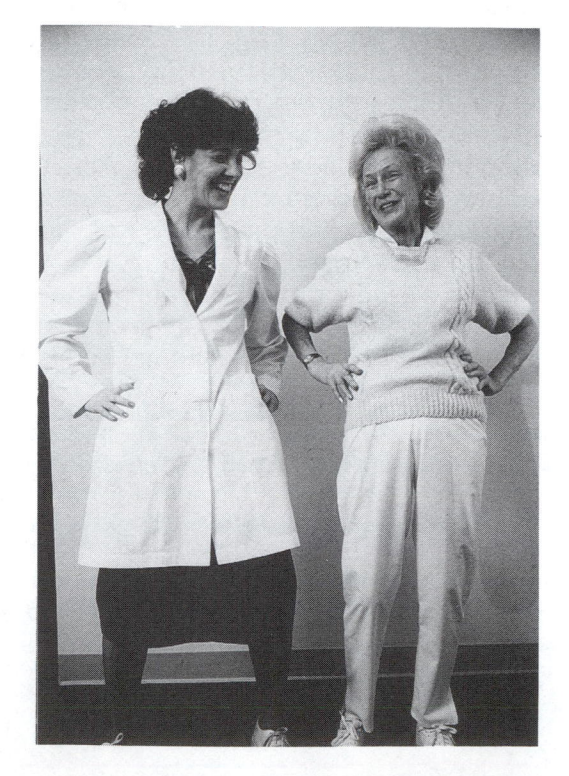

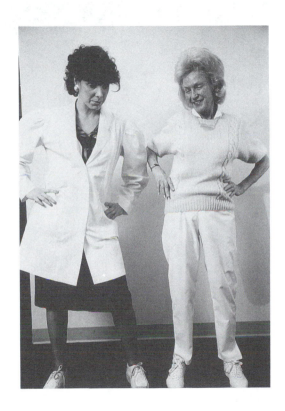

walk, feeling the air, the floor, and the muscle movement in detail. When they actually do the walking, certain training programs can be helpful. For example, the rehabilitation specialist may encourage weight shift instead of trunk lurch when hip abductors are weak. The patient will almost be "ice skating" (Figure 6-3). The rehabilitation specialist may also break the gait pattern down into various parts and train activities in the component parts (Figure 6-4).

The sensory environment is extremely important. A person in the dark walks very differently from a person in a well-lit room, for example. Therefore, the rehabilitation specialist should make sure the lighting is adequate for patients to see what they are doing and where they are going.

Various ambulatory aids are available for patients with gait problems.[15] Caution is required, however, to be sure that ambulatory aids are properly fitted and correctly used. They must not be used too frequently, as patients may become dependent on them. On the other hand, the correct device can often help patients walk independently.

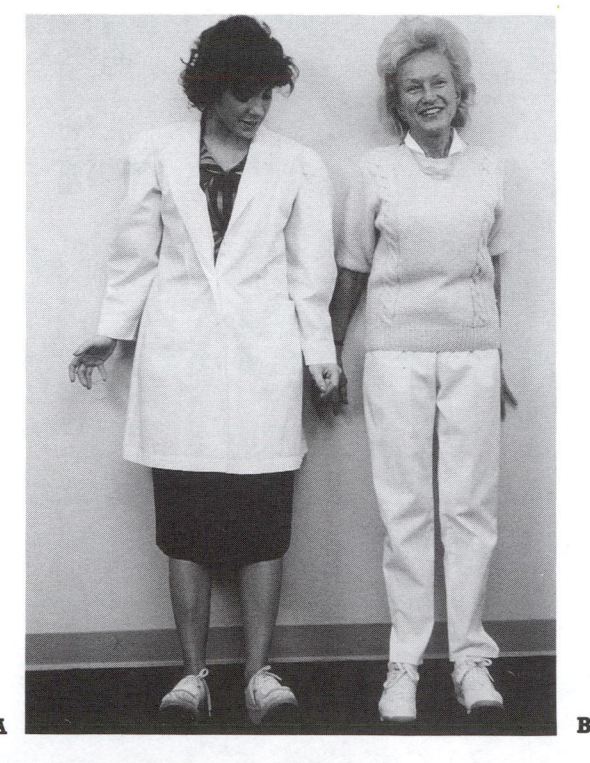

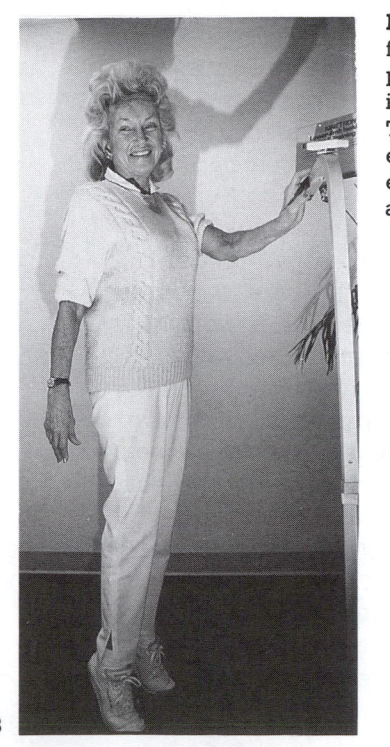

Figure 6-2 Gait Exercises **A.** Dorsiflexion Facilitation (Wall Flops). The person stands approximately 10 inches from the wall and falls back. This activity will elicit toe and ankle extension. **B.** Plantar flexion strengthening (Toe-ups). The person goes up and down on the toes.

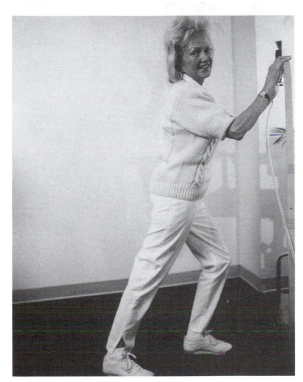

C. Hip and lower extremity stretches
Calf Stretch

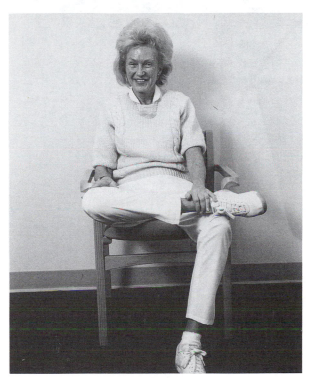

Hip Rotation Stretch

continues

D. Strengthening and facilitating terminal extension

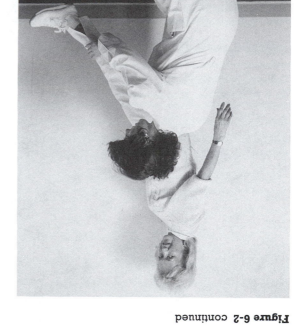

Figure 6-2 continued

E. Stretching hip abductors

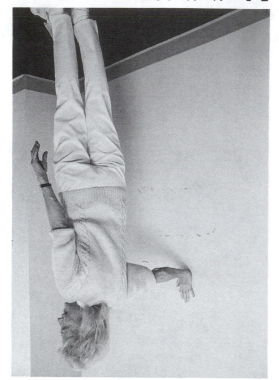

Figure 6-3 Facilitating Weight Shift While Walking

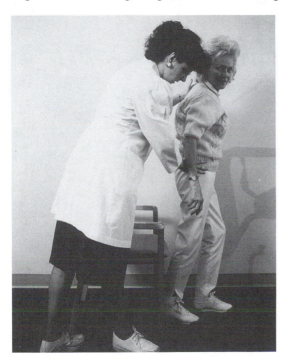

Figure 6-4 Gait Component Exercises

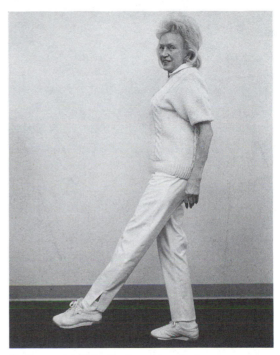

I. Leg swing (hip flexion extension)
    (standing leg swing, keeping trunk still)

continues

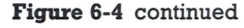

Figure 6-4 continued

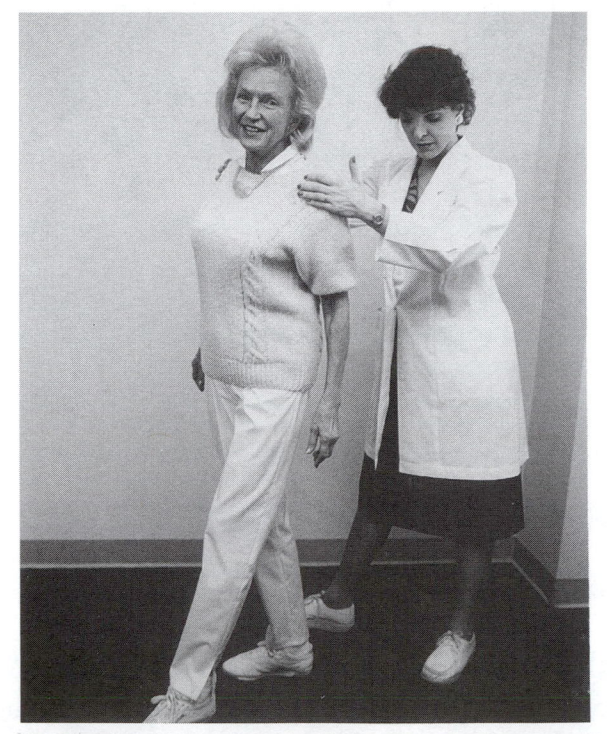

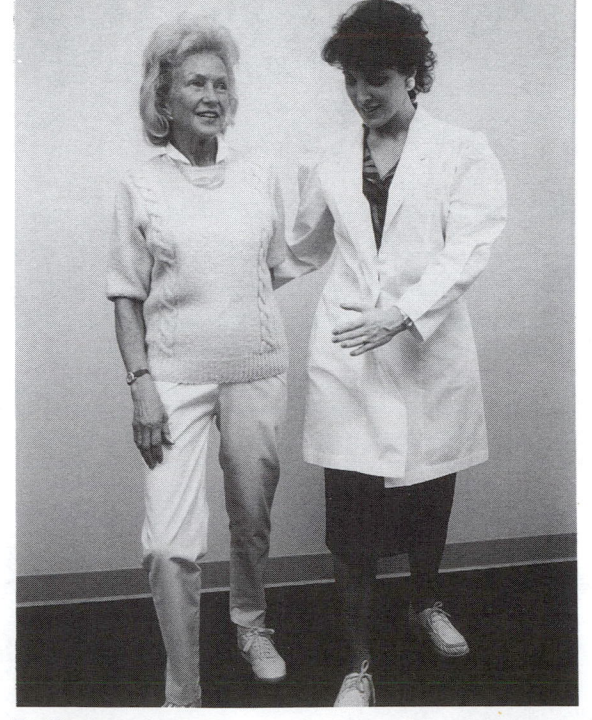

II. **A.** Toe off (toe-ups followed by heel cord stretch, **B.**)

B. Heel cord stretch

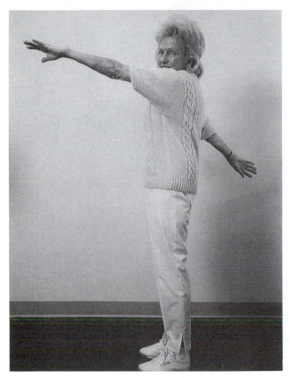

III. Arm swing (automatic movements) (practicing arm swing, then walking)

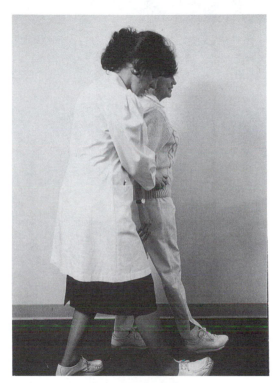

IV. Heel strike (practicing heel strike and weight acceptance)

continues

Figure 6-4 continued

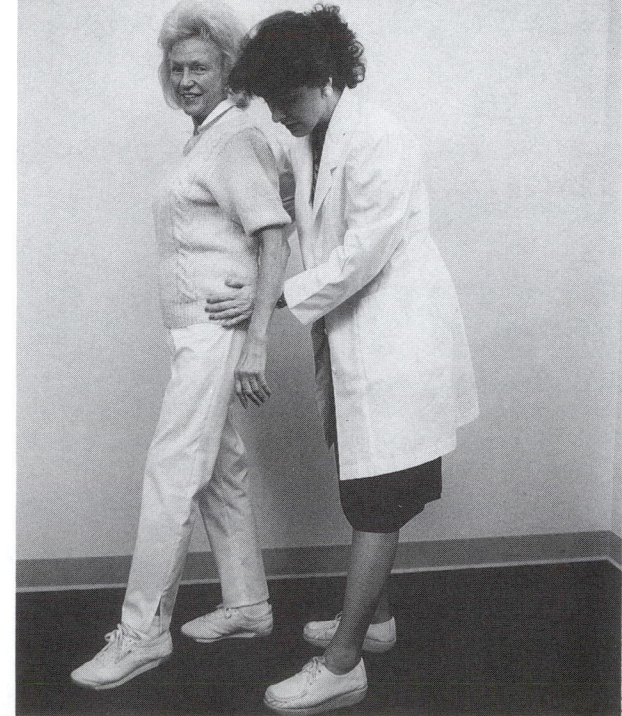

V. Rotating hip manually

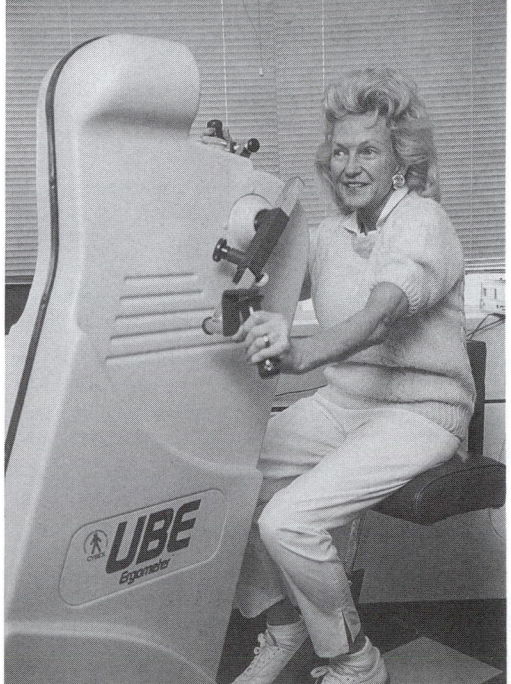

VI. Rotating trunk mechanically

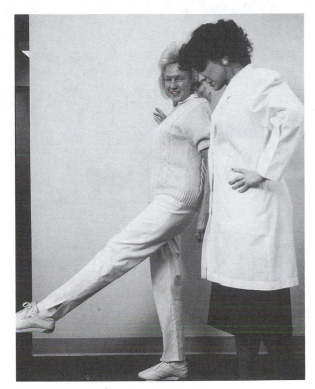

VII. Terminal extension. **A.** Standing

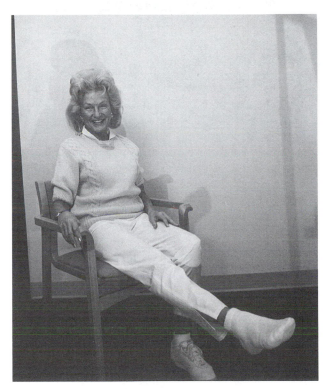

B. Sitting

continues

Gait

VIII. Hip flexion

C. Mechanically

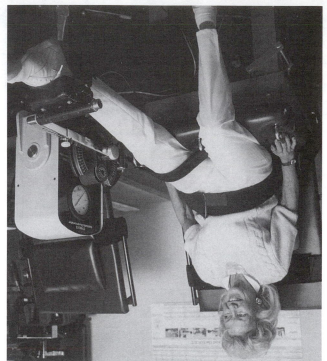

Figure 6-4 continued

COMMUNITY AMBULATION

In a study of community ambulators in Los Angeles, Frankel and his associates[16] found that independent community ambulators must walk over steps 10 inches high and must be able to walk approximately 300 meters to banks, stores, drug stores, or grocery stores. Therefore, those who plan to be community ambulators must do more than reach independence on flat surfaces at 50 feet in the rehabilitation process; in order to return to community life, they must become independent in several other parameters (Table 6-1).

The overriding considerations for the rehabilitation specialist are the requirements for walking:

- *The awareness of the need for action:* Does the patient want to get up and move?

- *The source of motion:* Does the patient have enough strength and flexibility to walk?

- *Cardiopulmonary status:* Does the patient have enough energy in the cardiopulmonary system to be able to walk?

Table 6-1 Characteristics of Community Ambulators. Mean Values—Distances, Curb Heights, Street Crossing Times

Destination	X	Range
	meters	*meters*
Crosswalk length (residential)	13	8–16
Crosswalk length (commercial)	27	22–34
Post Office	64	33–102
Bank	98	50–179
MD office	98	43–159
Supermarket	267	233–338
Department store	286	174–381
Drugstore	332	148–597
	cm	*cm*
Curb height (commercial)	20	15–22
Curb height (residential)	18	14–22
	seconds	*seconds*
Crosswalk time	20.5	16–23

Note: For the measurement of businesses and offices, the distance from the closest parking place to halfway through the ground floor of each establishment was used.

Source: Reprinted from *Clinical Management in Physical Therapy,* Vol. 6, No. 2, with permission of American Physical Therapy Association, © 1986.

- *Movement and control:* Does the patient's central nervous system function well enough to provide information for the use of the limbs? Does the patient have the appropriate proprioceptive information and the appropriate neuromusculature information?

If the answer to any of these questions is no, then the older person will have a more difficult time attaining independence in the next phase of the mobility spectrum: balance.

NOTES

1. D.A. Cunningham et al., "Determinants of Self Selected Walking Pace Across Ages 19 to 66," *Journal of Gerontology* 37 (1982): 560.
2. M.P. Murray, R.C. Kory, and B.H. Clarkson, "Walking Patterns in Healthy Old Men," *Journal of Gerontology* 24 (1969): 169.
3. M. O'Brien et al., "Temporal Gait Patterns in Healthy Young and Elderly Females," *Physiotherapy Canada* 35 (1983): 323.
4. R.D. Croninshield, R.A. Brand, and R.C. Johnston, "The Effects of Walking Velocity and Age on Hip Kinematics and Kinetics," *Clinical Orthopedics* 132: 14.
5. L. Sudarsky and M. Ronthal, "Gait Disorders Among Elderly Patients," *Archives of Neurology* 40 (1983): 740.
6. F.R. Findley, K.A. Coaly, and R.V. Fenizie, "Locomotion Patterns in Elderly Women," *Archives of Physical Medicine and Rehabilitation,* 50 (1967): 140.
7. Ibid.
8. T.P. Andriacchi, J.A. Ogle, and J.O. Galante, "Walking Speed as a Basis of Normal and Abnormal Gait Measurements," *Journal of Biomechanics* 10 (1977): 261.
9. Ibid.
10. Ibid.
11. R.L. Walters, J. Perry, and J.M. McDaniels, "The Relative Strength of the Hamstrings During Hip Extension," *Journal of Bone and Joint Surgery* 56A (1974): 1592.
12. J. Perry, "Integrated Function of the Lower Extremity Including Gait Analysis," in R.L. Cruess and W.R.J. Pennie, eds., *Adult Orthopedics* (New York: Churchill Livingstone, 1984), p. 1161.
13. A. Nelson, "Functional Ambulation Profile," *Physical Therapy* 54 (1974): 1061.
14. Ibid.
15. G. Pawlson and C. Lewis, "Dysmobility," in Karpan, ed., *Aging and Clinical Practice: Musculoskeletal Disorders: A Regional Approach* (New York: Igaku-Shoin, 1988).
16. B. Frankiel-Lerner et al., "Functional Community Ambulation: What Are Your Criteria," *Clinical Management* 6, no. 2 (1985): 37–41.

Balance

VII

Balance courses through all the upright postures and mobility steps. Thus, balance should be assessed not only when a person is standing and walking but as soon as the person sits up.

Balance has been defined as "the harmonious adjustments of parts and performance of functions."[1] In addition, it is the body's ability to function as a whole to create symmetry and ease of movement. It has several components and involves all the systems of the body. Therefore, in working with balance problems, it is imperative that the rehabilitation specialist take into account all the systems. The most effective treatment of a person with balance problems begins with a thorough medical screening by a geriatrician and a thorough evaluation by a rehabilitation professional.

SOURCES OF BALANCE PROBLEMS

Problems in balance may originate in any one of a variety of systems. Muscles that are weak, tight, or out of alignment contribute to balance problems. For example, weakness in the plantar flexors, dorsiflexors, quadriceps, and hamstring muscles strongly correlates with balance problems.[2] Tightness in the hip flexors, external rotators, plantar flexors, and knee flexors affect balance.[3] Alignment relates to the body's vertical position. If muscles are short or positioned at an abnormal angle, the body may tend to move in that direction, lose muscle advantage, and, hence, lose balance.

Some changes in the neurological system that occur with age affect balance. The older person has decreased reaction time, decreased proprioception at the foot, decreased vibratory sensation of the toes, and an increased sway pattern.[4,5] Older persons also have decreased stimulation of the receptors in the neck[6] and a significant decrease in vestibular sensory input.[7] Each of these factors can lead to problems with balance.

Woollacott, Shumway-Cook, and Nashner[8] found that people tend to lose the ability to choose the appropriate motor strategy when they get older. For example, if a person standing on a corner sees a bus go by, the visual cue suggests that the person is moving rather than the bus. The perceptual cues that the person was receiving from the feet tells the person that the bus is moving, not the person. If one followed the visual cues as one's balance strategy, one would probably fall forward. In other words, there is a conflict between a cue from the eyes and a cue from the feet. The older person is likely to take the wrong cue. In addition, older people have difficulty initiating motions[9] and coordinating the sequence of muscle activators required to compensate for the loss of balance.[10]

In the cardiovascular area, the vertebral artery syndrome may be responsible for loss of balance. With this syndrome, rotating and extending the neck prevents blood from reaching the brain and, as a result, causes the patient to lose his or her balance. This is due to the flattening of the cervical disc with age and the resultant tortuousness of the vertebral artery, which makes the artery more susceptible to occlusion by head movement (Figure 7-1).[11] Orthostatic hypotension, a condition in which the cardiovascular system is unable to adjust quickly enough to supply enough blood to the brain when a person stands up suddenly, may also be responsible for a loss of balance. Patients who are cardiovascularly deconditioned when they increase their activity level may lose their balance—again because of an inadequate blood supply to the body parts. A myocardial infarction may actually manifest itself as dizziness in older persons rather than the typical squeezing chest pain found in younger persons.[12]

The rehabilitation specialist should not overlook the psychological system as a cause for balance problems. Older people may be confused and may respond to the wrong balance cues in the environment. In addition, fear is a big problem for many older persons. Coining the term *ptophobia* (fear of falling), Bhala, O'Donnell, and Thoppil[13] described the anxiety reactions of older persons to the risk of falling. They urged rehabilitation specialists to screen their older patients for this problem. Finally, depression may interfere with balance. Depressed older persons may not be motivated or interested in walking or balance. They may not be

Figure 7-1 Vertebral Artery Syndrome.

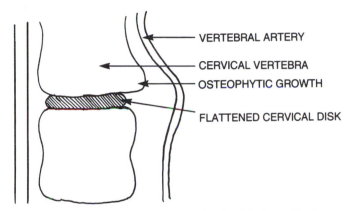

VERTEBRAL ARTERY

CERVICAL VERTEBRA

OSTEOPHYTIC GROWTH

FLATTENED CERVICAL DISK

Source: Reprinted from *Aging: The Health Care Challenge* by C.B. Lewis, p. 138, with permission of F.A. Davis Company, © 1985.

able to see any advantages to improving their balance.

EVALUATION OF BALANCE

A balance screening tool, such as that shown in Exhibit 7-1, may be used as an initial balance assessment form. Each item relates to a person's risk for a fall or a balance problem. Such a form cues the rehabilitation specialist to check for current medical problems, medications, and history of falls, as well as systemic causes of balance problems.

The rehabilitation specialist should have as much background information as possible on medical problems that may be contributing to balance problems. Inner ear disease, for example, may be the sole reason for balance problems and may not respond to rehabilitation efforts. Medications often affect balance, and the rehabilitation specialist should know what medications a patient is taking.

An investigation of earlier falls can provide a great deal of useful information. A history of frequent falls suggests neuromuscular or cardiovas-

Exhibit 7-1 Balance Screening Tool

```
  1. Name _____
  2. Date _____
  3. Current medical problems _____
  4. Medications _____
  5. History of falls _____
       Frequency _____
       Time of day _____
       Position _____
       Activity _____
       Circumstances _____
  6. Balance with eyes open _____
  7. Balance with eyes closed _____
  8. Balance right _____ Eyes closed _____
  9. Balance left _____ Eyes closed _____
 10. Push balance recovery _____
 11. Get up and go _____
 12. Balance actuator _____
 13. Vertebral Artery Syndrome _____
 14. Lying to sitting _____
 15. Sitting to standing _____
 16. Flexibility _____
 17. Strength _____
 18. Posture _____
 19. Gait _____ Eyes closed _____
 20. Tandem walk _____
 21. Psychological _____
 22. Comments _____
```

cular complications. Time of day suggests cardio-vascular deconditioning or psychological complications. Information on position may reveal orthostatic hypotension. Asking the patient to reenact a fall reveals a great deal about the circumstances.

In order to check the patient's balance with the eyes open, the rehabilitation specialist simply asks the patient to stand and then examines the sway pattern. Then the rehabilitation specialist repeats the procedure with the patient's eyes closed to determine whether the sway increases with closed eyes. Similarly, the rehabilitation specialist assesses the patient's balance on each leg with the patient's eyes open and with the patient's eyes closed. Bohannon et al.[14] found that there was a significant decrease in an older person's standing balance when the eyes were closed.

In order to determine the patient's push balance recovery (Figure 7-2), the rehabilitation specialist has the patient stand, gently pushes the patient's sternum, and assesses the patient's response. The rehabilitation specialist should note whether the patient makes a total body response, gently falls back, or responds slowly.

Figure 7-2 Push Balance Recovery

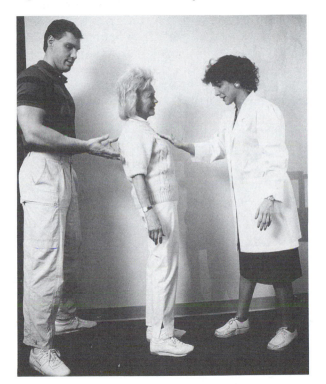 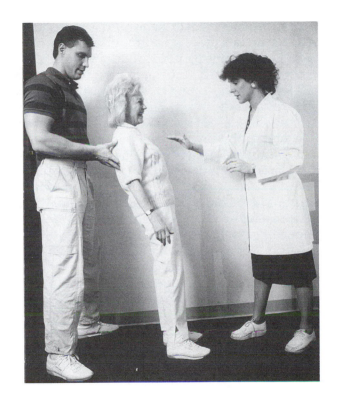

For the get-up-and-go test, the rehabilitation specialist asks the patient to sit, rise, stand, walk 3 meters, turn, walk back, and sit.[15] The patient's performance is rated on a scale of 0 to 5:

- 1, no evidence or risk of fall
- 2, moderately abnormal
- 3, mildly abnormal
- 4, very slightly abnormal
- 5, severely abnormal, risk of fall

This test correlated very strongly with balance problems and falling.

An instrument called a "balance actuator" may be used to assess balance (see Chapter 10). The patient tries to balance on a board while the actuator automatically measures shifts in weight and changes in balance (Figure 7-3). The balance actuator indicates the number of seconds the patient touches on one side and the number of weight shifts. One study[16] in which the balance actuator was used with both younger and older patients showed that the older group tended to have fewer touches but longer times at each touch.

To be screened for the vertebral artery syndrome, patients lie down and put their neck into extension and rotation to determine if they become nauseated, get dizzy, or develop nystagmus. If they do, this may be a positive indication for vertebral artery syndrome. This can mean that they will have balance problems if they turn their head and extend their neck.

Positionally related balance problems are checked by having the patient go from lying to sitting and sitting to standing and determining dizziness in each maneuver.

Flexibility, especially of the lower extremities (muscles, hip flexors, rotators, knee flexors, and extensor and plantar flexors), can be checked easily by range of motion and strength lists. Strength in the lower extremities should be tested to discover any abnormalities that may cause asymmetries or loss of balance. Proprioceptive difficulties may be revealed by having patients walk in tandem or march with their eyes closed.

Figure 7-3 Balance Actuator

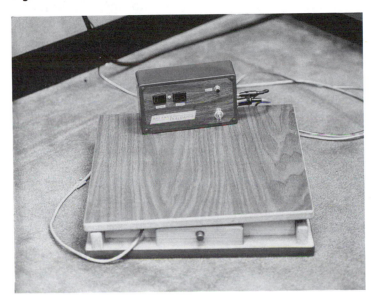

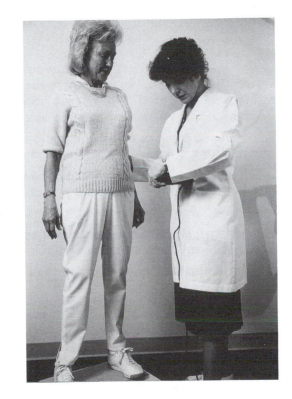

Finally, the rehabilitation specialist should note any comments about fear or sadness.

TREATMENT PROGRAMS FOR BALANCE PROBLEMS

The thorough evaluation of the patient's balance problems determines the appropriate treatment program. If, for example, muscle tightness was noted, it would be necessary to work on specific stretching exercises and to incorporate such exercises into a daily activity. If the problem is neurological, the patient would need training in proprioception (e.g., walking on various pieces of foam or thick carpeting) or compensation techniques (Figure 7-4) (e.g., using other senses to overcome the loss of proprioception). If the problem is cardiovascular, the rehabilitation specialist would teach the patient how to move from sitting to standing and from standing to sitting by resting and counting until he or she felt stable. It is helpful if the patient makes this a habit.

The rehabilitation specialist should provide positive suggestions to help patients gain confidence.

Realistic reinforcement has been shown to help depressed persons. For patients with a fear of falling, the treatment is:

- to keep them in familiar surroundings
- to shape their behavior progressively (take small progressive steps toward each goal)
- to treat them frequently
- to provide walking aids, but gradually eliminate those aids
- to make sure they master their current level before progressing to the next level
- to use contact desensitization, touching them a great deal at first, then less as they become more stable, less fearful, and more independent [17]

If a patient has a vestibular problem, the vestibular system can be stimulated by rocking, as well as by other activities performed in a seated position.[18] The autonomic nervous system interventions

Figure 7-4 Compensation Techniques

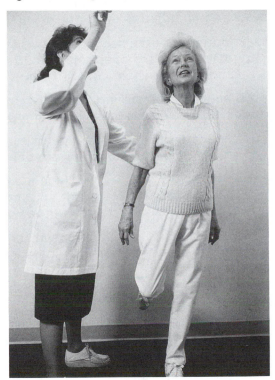

A. One-legged standing looking in different directions

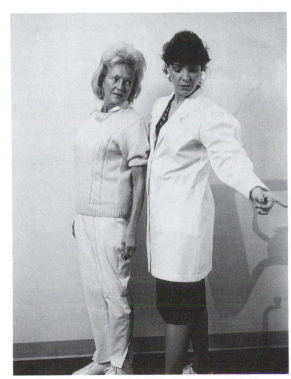

B. Two-legged standing with cervical rotation

mentioned in terms of transfer activities can be beneficial for those with balance problems (see Chapter 4). Finally, general balance hints can be helpful to patients:

- Maintain an adequate base of support (feet slightly apart).

- Lower the center of gravity when greater stability is needed (crouch when a fall is imminent).

- Keep the line of gravity within the base of support; stand with proper body alignment.

- Widen the base of support in the direction of the force; for example, lean into the wind.

- Increase friction between the body and the supporting surface for better stability; wear rubber-soled shoes for better gripping action.

- Maintain adequate strength in the legs to provide the force necessary to regain balance after unexpected loss.

- Focus vision on stationary objects rather than on moving objects.

- Practice mentally.

In the area of mental practice, ideokinetic facilitation has been shown to produce tremendous results.[19] People in one study who visualized for 30 minutes, three times a week, dramatically improved their balance. They were given the following instructions:

Now think about balancing. Remember what it was like to play balancing games as a child. Remember how easy it was to stand on one leg. Remember how long you could balance playing hopscotch. Remember how easy and fun it was to walk along a thin wall.

Think about your balance now. Realize that the balance you had as a child is still yours. You can balance, you just need to practice and to remind yourself of how easy it can be.

As you stand on one leg, see yourself as a tall oak tree. Feel the support of the roots beneath you. Feel your arms like branches, reaching out to the sky, helping to support you in the air. Enjoy the feeling of standing calm and still in the wind.

See a large brightly colored bird. Imagine you are that bird. You have long, strong legs. You lift up one leg and begin to balance. Feel how securely you stand and begin to balance. Feel how securely you stand on one leg with the other tucked comfortably up beneath you.*

Like all the components of the mobility spectrum, balance is a complicated process. Sharp investigative and integrative strategies are required to overcome problems. Older persons who have balance problems must be encouraged to continue a program, as the benefits of a program may not be immediately apparent.

*Reprinted from *Physical Therapy,* Vol. 65, p. 1338, with permission of American Physical Therapy Association, © 1985.

NOTES

1. *Dorland's Illustrated Medical Dictionary,* 124th ed. (Philadelphia: W.B. Saunders, 1965), p. 178.

2. R. Whipple, L. Wolfson, and P. Amerman, "The Relationship of Knee and Ankle Weakness to Falls in Nursing Home Residents: An Isokinetic Study," *Journal of the American Geriatric Society* 35, no. 1 (1987): 1.

3. Ibid.

4. R. Katzman and R.D. Terry, "Normal Aging of the Nervous System," in R. Katzman and R.D. Terry, eds., *The Neurology of Aging* (Philadelphia: F.A. Davis, 1983), p. 15.

5. P.W. Overstall, A.L. Johnson, and A.N. Exton-Smith, "Instability and Falls in the Elderly," *Age and Aging* Supp. 7 (1978): 92.

6. B. Wyke, "Cervical Articular Contributions to Posture and Gait: Their Relation to Senile Disequilibrium," *Age and Aging* 8 (1979): 251.

7. C.E. Stelmach and C.J. Worringham, "Sensorimotor Deficits Related to Postural Stability: Implications for Falling in the Elderly," *Clinics in Geriatric Medicine* 1, no. 3 (Aug., 1985): 679–695.

8. A. Shumway-Cook and F.B. Horak, "Assessing the Influence of Sensory Interaction on Balance," *Physical Therapy* 66 (1986): 1548.

9. M.H. Woollacott, A. Shumway-Cook, and L.M. Nashner, "Postural Reflexes and Aging," in J.A. Mortimer, F.J. Pirozzalo, and A.J. Malletta, eds., *The Aging Motor System* (New York: Praeger Publishers, 1982), p. 98.

10. M.H. Woollacott, A. Shumway-Cook, and L.M. Nashner, "Aging and Posture Control," *International Journal of Aging and Human Development* 23 (1986): 97; R. Wooton, E.

Bryon, U. Elarris, H. Greeman, J.R. Green, and R. Hesp. "Risk Factors for Fractured Neck of Femur in the Elderly," *Age and Aging* 11 (1982): 160.

11. M. Louis. "Falls and Their Causes." *Journal of Gerontological Nursing* 9 (1983): 142

12. D. Tresch, "Atypical Presentation of Cardiovascular Disorders in the Elderly," *Geratrics* 42, no. 10 (1987): 31–37.

13. R. Bhala, J.E. O'Donnell, and Thoppil. "Ptophobia: Phobic Fear of Falling and Its Clinical Management," 62, no. 2 (1982): 197–198.

14. R.W. Bonannon et al., "Decreased in Timed Balance Test Scores With Aging," *Physical Therapy* 64 (1984): 1067.

15. S. Mathias, L. Rayak, and B. Isaacs, "Balance in Elderly Patients: Get-up and Go Test," *Archives of Physical Medicine and Rehabilitation* 67 (1986): 387.

16. K. Schaefer and C. Lewis, "Balance Actuator Assessment." Physical Therapy Services of Washington, D.C., Inc. (1987).

17. S. Herdman, "Patients with Vestibular Disorders," *Postgraduate Advances in Physical Therapy* (Alexandria, Va.: Forum Medicus and the American Physical Therapy Association: 1987), pp. 1–12.

18. Ibid.

19. L.C. Fansler, C.L. Poff, and K.F. Shepard, "Effects of Mental Practice on Balance in Elderly Women," *Physical Therapy* 65, no. 9 (1985): 1332–1336.

Sensory Environment

VIII

The major senses, particularly hearing and vision, have a great impact on dysmobility and rehabilitation progress. Hearing loss affects 30 to 60 percent of persons over the age of 61.[1] Eighty percent of people over the age of 65 need glasses to be independent in daily activities, and 46 percent of the legally blind are over the age of 65.[2] These sensory deficits probably occurred very slowly, so slowly that the decreased information obtained through the senses and the concomitant decreased ability to assess the environment accurately may not even have been noticed. A difference in various activities, however, was noticed.

AGE-RELATED CHANGES IN THE SENSES

The prefix *presby,* meaning old age, occurs frequently in any discussion of sensory changes with age. *Presbycusis,* the uniform and irreversible decrease in the ability to hear high-frequency sounds, is the change in hearing that occurs in old age. People in high-noise areas have a greater hearing loss than do people in low-noise areas. Problems associated with presbycusis include the following:

- The person may not be sure where sounds are coming from, especially in a group setting. Treatment suggestion: distinguish visually who is speaking, e.g., person holds gavel or Nerf ball.

- The inability to hear consonants makes it difficult to understand sentences. Treatment suggestion: enunciate consonants and speak slowly and clearly.

- The sound range is reduced, and sounds outside the range may be irritating. Treatment suggestion: watch for looks of irritation and lower or raise the sound accordingly.

- Competing noises (e.g., conversation or background music) may be heard more clearly than the primary sound. Treatment suggestion: avoid extraneous background conversation and music; have a room set aside that is quiet.

- High tones may be irritating; the person may prefer lower tones in music and voices. Treatment suggestion: lower the voice and set the music on bass tones.

- Sounds at some frequencies, such as those associated with crushing leaves or an oncoming bicycle, may not be heard at all. Treatment suggestion: teach the person to look for environmental cues and learn other ways to compensate.

- Some older persons may avoid interaction because their hearing is so poor. Treatment suggestion: encourage these people to be involved by using extra nonverbal communication.

- Persons may hear selectively. Because hearing correctly can be a chore, they may decide not to bother. Treatment suggestion: be aware of this behavior, be patient, and use this information to determine person's priority for the message.

Presbyopia, or old age blindness, has the following problems associated with mobility:

- Similar colors appear the same. An older person may not be able to distinquish floors from chairs that are of the same color. Treatment suggestion: use contrasting colors or tape to set apart similar colors.

- A person going into a bright area after being in a darker one may be blinded by the glare and lose physical orientation. Treatment suggestion: do not use high-gloss floor wax and avoid shiny floors, windows, and upholstery. The person should use sunglasses and a hat when going out on a sunny day.

- The lens of the eye becomes thicker with age, and the person needs more light to see correctly. Treatment suggestion: use a lot of light

(200 watts), especially in functional areas (e.g., reading spots, kitchens, and bathrooms).

EVALUATION OF THE SENSORY ENVIRONMENT

A general and quick evaluation can reveal problem areas in the sensory environment. Each area in the environment should be carefully assessed to ensure that it is safe for the patient with a sensory deficit (Exhibit 8-1). Many institutions have specific evaluation forms that they use in their efforts to make the environment much safer for the sensorily impaired older person (Exhibit 8-2). Various home assessment tools are also available (Exhibit 8-3).

TREATMENT STRATEGIES

There are several techniques that may be used to compensate for sensory problems. The following suggestions are helpful for those with hearing problems:

1. Speak slowly and clearly but do not shout.
2. Face the person at eye level so he or she can read your lips.
3. Lower the pitch of your voice if the hearing loss is in the high frequencies.
4. Adjust electronic or audio systems so that the bass or lower tones are predominant.
5. Avoid background noise whenever possible. Choose a quiet environment.
6. Check to see if the person's hearing aid is on and adjusted properly.
7. Use nonverbal communication in your conversations, such as smiles, waving, pointing, etc., to emphasize your "message."
8. Write a message that needs clarification.
9. Share in activities that require less pressure to communicate, such as cards, bowling, etc.
10. Orient the person about the topics of conversations which he or she cannot hear. This reduces the tendency to become paranoid or withdrawn.
11. Recognize that a hearing aid does not work for all people.

Exhibit 8-1 General Evaluation of the Sensory Environment

Name _____

Place _____

Date _____

Vision

Color contrasting _____

Food _____ Table _____ Plates _____

Pills _____

Rugs, floors, chairs _____

Stairs _____ Doorways _____

Glare

Windows _____

Floors _____

Furniture _____

Night lighting _____

Reading material _____

Lighting _____

Aids _____

Hearing

The person

Aids _____ Motivation _____

Vision _____ Stress _____

Skills _____ Social activities _____

Exhibit 8-2 Institutional Environmental Evaluation

	Yes	No
Lighting Does each room have multiple sources of light?		
Is the lighting diffuse?		
Is the lighting sufficiently bright?		
Are there blinds, drapes, sheer curtains across windows through which bright light shines?		
Are mirrors placed so that they do not reflect blinding amounts of light?		
Are older people seated so that bright soures of light are to their side?		
Colors Do wall colors contrast with the colors of floors and rugs?		
Are the predominant colors red, orange, pink, and yellow?		
Are blues and greens intense rather than pale?		
Are colors used to mark the edges of steps, curbs?		
Do small rugs contrast sharply in color with the floor?		
Is the paper used in making announcements, pamphlets, etc., a beige, off-white, yellow, or other warm color?		

Exhibit 8-2 continued

Lettering		
Are rooms, offices, signs, elevators, mailboxes, menus, notices, schedules, and so on, marked with sufficiently large and well-spaced lettering?		
Are letters and numbers in sharp contrast to their background?		
Is the print easy to read for the older person?		
Are the markings on appliances easily discerned, such as OFF/ON, or HOT/COLD?		
Are personal letters to older people written in large, legible script or in large type?		
Hearing Environment		
Is background noise reduced as much as possible?		
Are frequent interruptions by phones, people, or noises minimized?		
Are rooms adequately sound-proofed to facilitate conversation?		
Are conversational areas separated from areas containing noise-generating equipment?		
Communication		
Are your voice tones moderate?		
Do you avoid shouting?		
Is your speech moderate in pace?		
Do you enunciate your words?		
Do you directly face older people and catch their attention?		
Do you inform the hard-of-hearing person of changes in conversation?		

Are you seated within 3 to 5 feet of the older person?		
Are children instructed about ways of interacting with older people?		
Are phone amplifiers available?		
Are receivers available in public halls, churches, etc?		
Is adequate lighting available for the older person to see lips and facial expressions?		
Touch Does the environment contain a rich variety of textures that are easily accessible for the older person to feel?		
Does the environment contain a rich variety of objects that are interesting to touch?		
Do you and others shake hands warmly with older persons being welcomed into your setting?		
Do you know what forms of touch are appreciated by older persons with whom you interact?		
Dangerous Areas Are the edges of individual steps marked with a bright, contrasting color?		
Are protrusions on walls or floors carefully marked?		
Are curbs and driveways clearly marked?		
Are kitchen appliances, showers, baths, and so on, clearly marked as to ON/OFF or HOT/COLD positions?		

Source: Adapted from *The Sixth Sense,* The National Council on Aging, Washington, D.C., 1985.

Exhibit 8-3 Home Assessment Checklist for Fall Hazards

Exterior
- Are step surfaces nonslip?
- Are step edges visually marked to avoid tripping?
- Are steps in good repair?
- Are stairway handrails present? Are handrails securely fastened to fittings?
- Are walkways covered with a nonslip surface and free of objects that could be tripped over?
- Is there sufficient outdoor lighting to provide safe ambulation at night?

Interior
- Are lights bright enough to compensate for limited vision? Are light switches accessible to the patient before entering rooms?
- Are lights glare free?
- Are stairways adequately lighted?
- Are handrails present on both sides of staircases?
- Are handrails securely fastened to walls?
- Are step edges outlined with colored adhesive tape and slip resistant?
- Are throw rugs secured with nonslip backing?
- Are carpet edges taped or tacked down?
- Are rooms uncluttered to permit unobstructed mobility?
- Are chairs throughout home strong enough to provide support during transfers? Are armrests present on chairs to provide assistance while transferring?
- Are tables (dining room, kitchen, etc) secure enough to provide support if leaned on?
- Do low-lying objects (coffee tables, step stools, etc) present a tripping hazard?
- Are telephones accessible?

Kitchen
- Are storage areas easily reached without having to stand on tiptoe or a chair?
- Are linoleum floors slippery?

- Is there a nonslip mat in the sink area to soak up spilled water?
- Are chairs wheelfree, armrest equipped, and of the proper height to allow for safe transfers?
- If the pilot light goes out on the gas stove, is the gas odor strong enough to alert the patient?
- Are step stools strong enough to provide support? Are stool treads in good repair and slip resistant?

Bathroom
- Are doors wide enough to provide unobstructed entering with or without a device?
- Do door thresholds present tripping hazards?
- Are floors slippery, especially when wet?
- Are skid-proof strips or mats in place in the tub or shower?
- Are tub and toilet grab bars available? Are grab bars securely fastened to the walls?
- Are toilets low in height? Is an elevated toilet seat available to assist in toilet transfers?
- Is there sufficient, accessible, and glare-free light available?

Bedroom
- Is there adequate and accessible lighting available? Are night-lights and/or bedside lamps available for nighttime bathroom trips?
- Is the pathway from the bed to the bathroom clear to provide unobstructed mobility (especially at night)?
- Are beds of appropriate height to allow for safe on and off transfers?
- Are floors covered with a nonslip surface and free of objects that could be tripped over?
- Can patient reach objects from closet shelves without standing on tiptoe or a chair?

Source: Reprinted from *Topics in Geriatric Rehabilitation,* Vol. 3, No. 1, p. 59, Aspen Publishers, Inc., © October 1987.

12. Remember that what appears to be "selective hearing" may actually be due to factors such as high frequency, fatigue, and environmental distractions.*

In addition, it is helpful to make it possible for the hearing-impaired person to distinguish visually who is speaking (e.g., the person holding a ball). Other suggestions for visually impaired persons are:

1. Provide adequate light. Persons with visual problems need much more light than the average person.
2. Reduce glare. Avoid shiny surfaces which will reflect light. Window shades, blinds, sunglasses, visors or hats with brims may reduce the glare from sunlight.
3. Avoid color coding when safety is a factor. Pastel colors, blues, greens, and very dark colors may all look alike to the elderly. Color coding should not be used for pills, markings on appliances, etc. Colors used for identification and location should be strongly contrasting, such as yellow and blue.
4. Avoid abrupt changes in light. The older eye takes more time to accommodate to sudden changes. Lights should be strategically arranged, and some lights should be kept on at night in hazardous locations. For example, night lights can be left on in the bedroom, hall, and bath so there is an even distribution of light.
5. Use large print on all signs, directions, labels, etc. Large print is easier for everyone to see.
6. People with cataract lenses may need assistance crossing streets or wherever depth perception is a safety factor.
7. Low vision aids, such as large print books, magnifying glasses, etc., may be of assistance.
8. Touching can be used in communication when vision is limited. A pat on the hand can let someone know you are listening.
9. Verbally describe a new room or situation to a visually impaired person. Help him or her to

*Reprinted with permission from *An Introduction to Aging—Module I* by G.H. Maguire, p. 31, Howard University, Washington, D.C., 1982.

locate hazards, furniture, and who is in the room. Stay with him or her until he or she is comfortably oriented.*

The literature contains a great deal of practical information on ways that rehabilitation specialists can help the patient compensate for sensory loss. Environmental safety is a matter of screening the environment to ensure an optimal environment for older persons with sensory loss.

COMMUNICATION AND TREATMENT OF MOBILITY PROBLEMS

In treating mobility problems in patients who have a sensory deficit, rehabilitation specialists must take the sensory deficit into account. In addition to the sensory loss, other aspects of communication should be considered. The following 14 communication strategies may be helpful in the mobility training of persons with sensory loss or psychological complications:

1. Try to supplement verbal comments with nonverbal cues. Use body language (e.g., hands and facial expressions).
2. Always use a surname when talking to older patients unless they ask otherwise. This shows respect.
3. Use a slow and clear tone when working with patients.
4. Use a call to action. Do not ask patients to do something, instead encourage them to do something: "Mrs. Jones, please stand up," not "Mrs. Jones, will you stand?"
5. Create a supportive visual environment. For example, the presence of a big sturdy chair often encourages a person to stand up even though he or she is afraid.
6. Use props that are attractive and motivating. For example, a colorful quilt draped over the chair or in the wheelchair to which a patient is transferring may encourage movement.

*Reprinted with permission from *An Introduction to Aging—Module I* by G.H. Maguire, p. 28, Howard University, Washington, D.C., 1982.

7. If the patient's response is very slow, build up the response time. For example, a patient with Parkinson's disease may need to start a movement by counting: "Ready, we are going to stand up, one, two, three, stand up" (to build up to the final command).
8. When directional instructions are nebulous (e.g., "lean forward"), use something more vivid (e.g., "nose over the toes" or "shoulders over the hips") to help the patient understand what specific body parts need to be in what place.
9. When a patient cannot respond on a cortical level to an instruction, such as "turn around," focus on the end of the task, not the task itself. Say, for example, "Come sit by your wife," or "Let's go to the window."
10. Reinforce instructions with sound cues. In helping a patient to sit on a chair, for example, hit the chair so that the patient hears and will know to go in the direction of the chair from the bed.
11. With fearful patients, try to keep the conversation going. For example, "I will help you." "I am going to bend your knees, I am going to move your leg, I am going to lift your left leg in the air." Say something to keep the patient involved throughout the therapy.
12. Do not let the patient fail more than once in a treatment session. Make sure that any failure is followed immediately by a success.
13. Use sensory cues. If a patient does not lean forward, for example, encourage the patient to lean forward by having him or her rub the thighs, then the knees, and eventually the calves.
14. Reassure any visual deficits. For example, when walking with patients who have a visual impairment, tell them that the floor is flat or that the carpet is thick in order to keep them aware of their environment.

The rehabilitation specialist must be aware of the importance of the sensory environment for mobility. It is essential to be open to creative ways of compensating for visual, hearing, and psychological deficits.

NOTES

1. National Council on Aging, *The Sixth Sense* (Washington, D.C.: 1985).
2. G. Maguire, "The Changing Realm of the Senses," in C. Lewis, ed., *Aging Health Cares Challenge Interdisciplinary Assessment and Treatment* (Philadelphia: F.A. Davis, 1983), pp. 101–116.

Drugs IX

Drugs can affect mobility positively or negatively. For example, L-dopa can help a patient with Parkinson's disease move better; on the other hand, this same drug can cause postural hypotension and, therefore, place the patient at risk for a fall. The rehabilitation specialist should be aware of the older person's altered response to drugs and the effects of various drugs on mobility.

DRUG-TAKING BEHAVIOR OF THE ELDERLY

The older population is at a greater risk for drug problems than is any other segment of the population because they take more drugs than does any other segment of the population, both prescription drugs[1] and over-the-counter drugs.[2] They are also known for being "pill swappers." Many studies have shown that drug takers have an increased tendency to fall.[3-5] Moreover, the more drugs taken, the greater the risk for falls.[6] As those who have multiple illnesses tend to take more drugs and as the older population has more illnesses than does any other segment of the population, the implications are clear.

Older persons may not comply with the instructions of their physician regarding the use of medications as well as younger persons do.[7] Because of their poorer vision, they are unable to see the directions as well;[8] because of their poorer hearing, they do not hear the directions from the physician as well.[9] In addition, some containers (e.g., child-proof containers) may be too difficult for persons with arthritis to open.[10] Adding to their difficulty in complying with instructions is the fact that older persons may have difficulty swallowing pills.[11] Finally, because they take more medicine, it is difficult for them to organize the multiple aspect of their drug-taking behavior.[12]

AGE CHANGES THAT CONTRIBUTE TO ALTERED DRUG EFFECTS

Drugs have different effects in older persons than in younger persons partly because of the older person's decreased drug and nutrient absorption.[13] This occurs for several reasons:

1. The diminished fluid volume in older persons' gastrointestinal tract makes it more difficult for their body to break down drugs.
2. When the patient is impaired, as is often the case with older persons, gastrointestinal blood flow drugs are not absorbed from the gastrointestinal system as quickly.
3. Because of diminished gastric acidity, it takes longer for drugs to break down in the older person's stomach.
4. There are fewer absorbing cells in the older person's gastrointestinal tract, which prolongs the process of drug absorption.
5. As a result of decreased gastric motility, drugs do not move through the older person's system as well.[14]

Not only the absorption but also the distribution of drugs are altered in the body of older persons.[15] Because older persons have less fluid in their system,[16] dissolving a drug in an older person's system produces a higher concentration than does dissolving the same amount of the drug in a younger person (Figure 9-1). Furthermore, there is a greater proportion of body fat in older persons, which means that the various fat-soluable drugs have a tendency to be stored in the fat.[17] Finally, the diminished plasma protein concentration in older persons may affect the binding of drugs at various protein binding sites.[18]

Drug metabolism is also altered in the elderly.[19] Because there is less hepatic enzyme activity to break down a drug,[20] the drug remains in the system longer. Moreover, hepatic blood flow is decreased in the elderly,[21] so the liver does not receive a blood supply adequate to break down the drug.

It is a well-documented fact that renal tubular function declines with age.[22,23] Therefore, the kidneys do not function as efficiently to excrete drugs.

Figure 9-1 Comparative Fluid Volumes

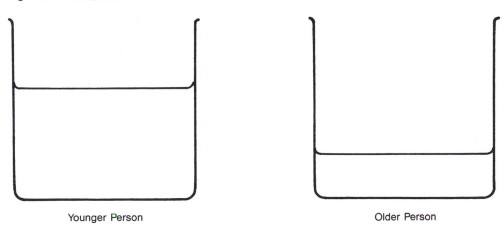

Younger Person   Older Person

Renal blood flow is decreased, which also affects the ability of the kidneys to excrete drugs.[24]

Certain other factors alter drug responses in the elderly. First, the presence of diseases has an impact on a drug's absorption.[25] When a person has a disease, the body may respond to certain drugs in unexpected ways. Second, altered receptor sensitivity can affect the manner in which a drug is absorbed. Third, and very important, an impaired homeostatic mechanism may decrease the ability of older persons to adjust to the environment and, thus, to the presence of a drug in their system.[26]

Nutritional and environmental factors may also alter drug effects in older persons. This segment of the population is known to be more poorly nourished than are other parts of the population,[27] and this poorer nutrition may affect the action of drugs.[28] Environmental factors can cause hyperthermia or hypothermia, which affects the ability of the body to absorb, metabolize, or excrete a drug.[29]

In treating an older person, the physician tries to prescribe medication in an amount that will keep the concentration in the body above the minimum effective dose but below the toxic level (Figure 9-2). Because the older person has decreased distribution, decreased absorption, and decreased metabolism, the drug may be in the system longer; however, the concentration in the body may well rise to the toxic range. It is difficult for the physician to determine exactly how long a drug will stay in a particular person's system; therefore, any time that an older person is taking a drug, has changed the drug because of an exercise program, or has altered the amount of drug taken, there may be a toxic reaction. The rehabilitation specialist must be aware of this.

Figure 9-2 Drug Disposition in Older Persons

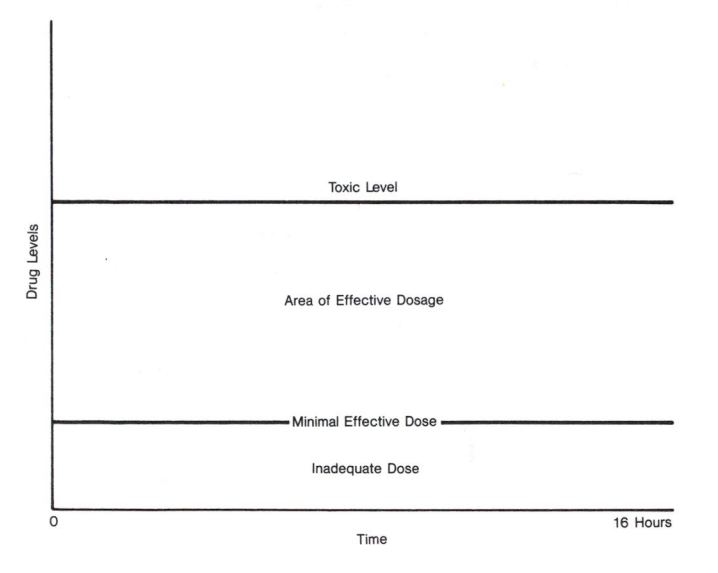

SPECIFIC TYPES OF DRUGS RELATED TO FALLS AND MOBILITY

Almost all types of drugs may affect mobility or the risk for falls (see Appendix C). Tranquilizers can cause generalized slowness and slight gait disturbances, for example.[30] Rehabilitation specialists should be aware of various tranquilizers that older persons may take if these symptoms and falls are a problem.

The following are other types of drugs that affect mobility:

- *Sedatives, hypnotics, and barbiturates:* Barbiturates have been directly linked to falls. In one study,[31] 93 percent of the people with hip fractures had been on barbiturates at the time of their fracture.

- *Tricyclic antidepressants:* These drugs have been known to cause postural hypertension, which can be a major cause of falls. Changes that occur in the baroreceptors with age alter the titration of various drugs. These drugs are difficult to titrate, a fact that may be responsible for the associated postural hypotension.[32]

- *Antihypertensives:* These drugs can cause postural hypotension, as well as weakness. The slightly decreased baroreflex sensitivity that occurs with age may cause problems when antihypertensives are administered. Older persons are especially prone to develop postural hypotension.[33]

- *Antiparkinsonism drugs:* These drugs can cause postural hypotension.

Because older people have less fluid volume; they can feel the effects of alcohol in their system sooner than younger persons can. Alcohol leads to increased sway and decreased visual input, which dramatically affect a person's ability to maintain balance and walk appropriately.

PATHOLOGY

As mentioned earlier, older persons have more illnesses than do other segments of the population.

It is important for the rehabilitation specialist to be aware of the most common illnesses, the drugs used to treat them, and their effect on dysmobility.

The most common medical problem in the older population is cardiovascular disease. Antihypertensive medications, if not administered appropriately, can cause dizziness or even hypotension. Some hypertensive medications, particularly nitrates and diuretics, can reach toxic levels because of the blood volume depletion in the older person. Beta blockers can also cause dizziness and lightheadedness. The side effects of inappropriate digoxin administration are dizziness, weakness, and vision change. Myocardial infarction may manifest as dizziness; this is a somewhat atypical symptom for a younger person, but rather typical (almost 38 percent) in older persons.[34]

In the psychosocial area, dysmobility may be caused by anxiety, depression, or dementia. For example, a depressed patient may not want to get up, or a demented patient may be slow or fatigued. Medications for these diseases can compound these symptoms. Tranquilizers and antidepressants, as well as some of the sedatives or antipsy-chotic drugs, can cause parkinsonism-like symptoms (e.g., bradykinesia and rigidity) that affect movement and function.[35]

Parkinsonism is very different from Parkinson's disease. There are many more patients with drug-induced parkinsonism than there are patients with Parkinson's disease. Patients with drug-induced parkinsonism can show postural instability, rigidity, bradykinesia, and resting tremors, although parkinsonism is more symmetrical than is Parkinson's disease. Because medication is directly linked to symptoms of parkinsonism, rehabilitation specialists who work on mobility problems with these patients may need to assess the timing of medication and programs and should directly consult the physician.[36]

The drug management of arthritis is relatively safe in terms of mobility problems. The only drugs known to cause problems are nonsteroidal anti-inflammatory drugs, which have a tendency to cause dizziness. Although no studies have shown a direct relationship between these drugs and a person's history of falling, rehabilitation specialists should be aware that drug management of arthritis can compound the immobility caused by the arthritis itself.[37]

In order to work best in the realm of drug interactions, rehabilitation specialists need to (1) be aware of the drugs most likely to be associated with falls; (2) recognize the diseases and drugs most likely to affect mobility; (3) have patients note the times of hypertension, dizziness, and vision change, and see if these correlate directly with the administration of drugs; (4) contact the physician to seek a change or a decrease in the medication; and (5) time therapy sessions to work most effectively with the patient's pharmaceutical management if severe drug problems occur regularly.[38]

NOTES

1. C. Baun et al., "Drug Use in the United States in 1981," *Journal of the American Medical Association* 251 (1984): 1293–1297.
2. F.E. Mary et al., "Prescribed and Nonprescribed Drug Use in an Ambulatory Elderly Population," *Southern Medical Journal* 75 (1982): 522.
3. A.M. Vener, S.R. Krupks, and J.J. Climo, "Drug Usage and Health Characteristics in Noninstitutionalized Retired Persons," *Journal of the American Geriatric Society* 27 (1979): 83.
4. R.B. Stewart et al., "Psychotropic Drug Use in an Ambulatory Elderly Population," *Gerontology* 28 (1983): 328.
5. F. Budden, "Adverse Drug Reactions in Long-Term Care Facility Residents," *Journal of the American Geriatric Society* 33 (1985): 449.
6. W. Simonson, *Medications and the Elderly* (Rockville, Md: Aspen Publishers, Inc. 1984), p. 7.
7. B. Blockwell, "Patient Compliance," *New England Journal of Medicine* 289 (1973): 299.
8. R.F. Gillum and A.J. Barsky, "Diagnosis and Management of Patient Noncompliance," *Journal of the American Medical Association* 228 (1974): 1563.
9. M.W. Gebhardt, J.F. Governali, E.J. Hart, "Drug Related Behavior: Knowledge and Misconceptions Among a Selected Group of Senior Citizens," *Journal of Drug Education* 8 (1978): 85.
10. Ibid.
11. C.I. Gryfe and B.M. Gryfe, "Drug Therapy of the Aged: The Problem of Compliance and the Roles of Physicians and Pharmacists," *Journal of the American Geriatric Society* 32 (1984): 301.
12. Ibid.
13. N. Horwitz, "Predisposing Factors in Adverse Reactions to Drugs," *British Medical Journal* 1 (1969): 536.
14. J.W. Smith, L.G. Seidl, and L.E. Cluff, "Studies on the Epi-

demiology of Adverse Drug Reactions: V. Clinical Factors Influencing Susceptibility," *Annals of Internal Medicine* 65 (1966): 65.

15. J.G. Wagner, "Biopharmaceutics: Absorption Aspects," *Journal of Pharmacological Science* 50 (1961): 359.

16. E. Kruger-Thiemer, "Dosage Schedules and Pharamacokinetics in Chemotherapy," *J. Am. Pharm. Assoc. Sci Ed.* 49 (1960): 311.

17. E. Nelson, "Kinetics of Drug Absorption, Distribution, Metabolism and Excretion," *Journal of Pharmacological Science* 50 (1961): 181.

18. Ibid.

19. R.E. Vestal and G.W. Dawson, "Pharmacology and Aging," in C.E. French and E.L. Schneider, eds., *Handbook of the Biology of Aging* (New York: Van Nostrand Reinhold, 1985), p. 771.

20. Ibid.

21. Ibid.

22. G.J. Greenblatt, E.M. Sellus, and R.I. Shader, "Drug Disposition in Old Age," *New England Journal of Medicine* 306 (1982): 1081.

23. Nelson, "Kinetics of Drug Absorption," 181.

24. Ibid.

25. Ibid.

26. Ibid.

27. Simonson, *Medications and the Elderly* (Rockville, Md.: Aspen Publishers, Inc., 1984), p. 7.

28. Ibid.

29. Ibid.

30. Ibid.

31. Ibid.

32. M.D. Blumenthal and J.W. Davie, "Dizziness and Falling in Elderly Psychiatric Outpatients," *American Journal of Psychiatry* 137 (1980): 203.

33. L.A. Lipsitz et al., "Postprandial Reduction in Blood Pressure in the Elderly," *New England Journal Of Medicine* 309 (1983): 81.

34. G.T. Kennedy and M.H. Crawford, "Optimal Positions and Timing of Blood Pressure and Heart Rate Measurements to Detect Orthostatic Changes in Patients with Ischemic Heart Disease," *Journal of Cardiac Rehabilitation* 4 (1984): 219.

35. Ibid.

36. M.H. Branchez et al., "High and Low-Potency Neuroleptics in Elderly Psychiatric Patients," *Journal of the American Medical Association* 239 (1978): 1860.

37. D. Chapron and R. Besdone, "Drugs: An Obstacle to Rehabilitation of the Elderly," *Topics in Geriatric Rehabilitation* 2, 3 (1987): 63–76.

38. R.G. Stewart, W.E. Hale, and R.G. Marks, "Analgesic Drug Use in an Ambulatory Elderly Population," *Clinical Pharmacology* 16 (1982): 833.

Resources X

This chapter is a listing of resources to enhance mobility for older persons. It may be used as a guide to new ideas and sources of information.

AUDIOVISUALS

Age Related Sensory Loss: An Empathetic Model
University of Michigan
Department of Gerontology
Ann Arbor, Michigan

This 25-minute videotape describes several aspects of presbyopia and presbycusis. The viewer can experience these losses by viewing a family dinner scene. Leo Pastalan, the narrator, is clear and concise in his presentation.

Armchair Fitness, by Betty Switkes
Productions, Inc.
P.O. Box 15707
Chevy Chase, MD 20815

This one-hour, fun to watch, exercise videotape demonstrates three exercise programs (20 minutes each). The first program is for beginners and the second and third programs are more advanced. Betty leads the class of seven various-aged participants. All are seated in a chair. The music, setting, and leader enthusiasm combine to make a very worthwhile tape.

At Home with Home Care
Billy Budd Films, Inc.
445 Main Street
Wyckoff, NJ 07481

This three-set videotape covers a diverse spectrum of topics related to caring for older persons in the home. A kindly nurse instructs a variety of family members on such topics as transferring, skin care, and exercise. Nine more topics are demonstrated on the tape. The tape is also easily indexed.

Increased Mobility for the Elderly, by the Rehabilitation Institute of Chicago

Aspen Publishers, Inc.
1600 Research Boulevard
Rockville, MD 20850

This long but thorough videotape describes the mobility limitation and interventions for three types of patients. Hands-on techniques are demonstrated for patients with Parkinson's disease, stroke, and arthritis. There is good introductory information about rehabilitation management.

Sixth Sense
The National Council on Aging
600 Maryland Avenue, S.W.
West Wing 100
Washington, DC 20024

This is an excellent and interesting tape depicting scenarios of sensory loss in different situations. The majority of the tape is short interviews with older persons and experts. The tape begins discussing aging and ends with graphic representations of hearing and vision loss.

Silver Foxes, by Richard Simmons
Karl-Lourimar Video Home, Inc.
17941 Cowen
Irvine, CA 92714

Richard Simmons, in his usual adorable manner, leads stars and parents through an exercise program. Almost all of the exercises are done standing and are very appropriate and fun for patients who can stand. The music and background encourage the viewer to exercise.

Senior Shape-Up Creative Fitness
Yablon Enterprises, Inc.
P.O. Box 7475
Steelton, PA 17113-0475

This 45-minute video tape is designed for sedentary and mildly active older persons. The exercises are clearly labeled and easy to understand and do. The music choice is excellent, using songs everyone should recognize.

Transfers: The Key to Independence for the Geriatric Bilateral Amputee
University of Maryland Physical School of Therapy
325 Greene Street
Baltimore, MD

This short but informative and emotion-packed video follows the life of an older man and woman who both live independently despite having bilateral amputations. Some basic information on transfer skills is discussed. The tape is an inspiring and motivating work.

Vitalife Videotapes
Vitalife Productions
14563 W. 96th Terrace
Lenexa, KS 66215
(913) 888-7304
$510 for a set of six, $88 per tape

This series of six outstanding videotapes covers information on multiple functional treatment problems relevant to caring for older persons. The six topics covered are:

1. activities of daily living
2. range of motion
3. transfer techniques
4. ambulation with assistance
5. protecting your back
6. positioning and turning

Each video tape is professional and of high quality. Each tape begins with introductory information on the topic provided in an interesting and fact-filled fashion by Fred Ward, a physical therapist. The introduction is followed by a comprehensive breakdown of the topic at hand. Ward not only gives the essential basic information, he also dots his presentation with information and animated anecdotes.

The tapes come with pause screens for reviewing purposes and a supplemental study guide. These clearly understood and easily reproducible booklets restate and test the important points of the video tapes.

Wheelercise, by Maura Casey
Scott & KC Enterprise, Inc.
P.O. Box 443
South Bound Brook, NJ 08880

Maura Casey, R.P.T., leads a healthy-looking group of wheelchair-bound individuals. The exercises are good but the setting and music are boring.

Walkerobics, by Maura Casey
Scott & KC Enterprise, Inc.
P.O. Box 443
South Bound Brook, NJ 08880

This is another video with Maura Casey and the boring gym and music. The tape does have some excellent exercises for patients at the walker level.

EQUIPMENT

Balance Actuator
Ohio Bio Medical Education Research
95 Park Lane
Mooreland Hills, OH 44022

This simple but easy to use electronic device measures a patient's static balance by electronically counting touches and time.

Back Supports
Medic-Air Back Support Pillows
Larchmont, NY 10538

These are inflatable pillows that can be used to support the lower back.

Foot Orthotics
Ali Med, Inc.
297 High Street
Dedham, MA 02026-2837

A variety of shoe molds and partial and full-foot orthotics are available from this company. This company also does free inservices on orthotic and shoe fabrication for older persons.

Posture Grid
Reedco
P.O. Box 345
51 North Fulton Street
Auburn, NY 13021

This 3 foot by 2 foot posture grid can hang from a doorway or wall. It provides horizontal and vertical lines as a backdrop for posture analysis.

Rehabilitation Xercise Bands™
SRI Products, Inc.
962 North Northwest Highway
Pork Ridge, IL 60068

These diverse bands provide graded resistance for exercising patients. These flat bands do not roll when a patient is exercising, and the different sizes provide graded resistance.

The Wedges (Ortho Leg Wedge & Cover, #9928)
Environment for Better Living
145 Tower Drive
P.O. Box 579
Hinsdale, IL 60521

Big and smaller wedges can be used for patient positioning.

Comfortably Yours (Bed Wedge, #L3053; Additional Cover, #L3054)
Aides for Easier Living
52 West Hunter Avenue
Maywood, NJ 07607

These wedges can be used for patient positioning to make patients more comfortable and pain free.

EVALUATION TOOLS

Ashworth Spasticity Scale
R. Bohannon and M. Smith, "Reliability of a Modified Ashworth Scale of Muscle Spasticity," *Physical Therapy* 67 (1986): 206.

This is a simple measure for spasticity. This scale has a relatively high reliability and validity.

Functional Independence Measure: Locomotion Scale
Task Force for Development of a Uniform Data System for Medical Rehabilitation Functional Independence (1986): 13.

This mobility measurement tool assesses grades of mobility independence. The directions, reliability, and validity of this tool are good.

Reedco Score Sheet
This provides a quick assessment tool for evaluating posture. The one-page grid evaluation has an interval scale ranking the components of posture by body part. Each ranking has a word and picture description. (See Figure 5-3.)

ORGANIZATIONS

Alzheimers Disease and Related Disorders Association
National Headquarters
70 Lake St.
Chicago, IL 60601

Arthritis Foundation
1901 Fort Meyer Drive
Suite 604
Arlington, VA 22207

National Council on the Aging, Inc.
1828 L Street, NW
Washington, D.C. 20036
(202) 223-6250

National Retired Teachers Association
1909 K Street, NW
Washington, D.C. 20005
(202) 872-4700

Parkinson Society
11376 Cherry Hill Road
Suite 204
Beltsville, MD 20705
(301) 937-1545

PROFESSIONAL ORGANIZATIONS WITH SPECIAL PROGRAM SECTIONS OR INTERESTS ON AGING

American Art Therapy Association
One Cedar Blvd.
Pittsburgh, PA 15228

American Association for Music Therapy
35 West Fourth Street
New York, NY 10003

American Association for Rehabilitation Therapy, Inc.
Box 93
North Little Rock, AR 72116

American Association for Respiratory Therapy
1720 Regal Row
Dallas, TX 75235
(214) 630-4700

American Association of Homes for the Aging
Suite 700
1050 17th Street, NW
Washington, D.C. 20036

American Association of Marriage and Family Counselors
225 Yale Avenue
Claremont, CA 91711

American Association of Physician Assistants
488 Madison Avenue
New York, NY 10022

American Association of Sex Educators and Counselors
5010 Wisconsin Avenue, NW
Washington, D.C. 20016

American College of Hospital Administrators
840 North Lake Shore Drive
Chicago, IL 60611

American College of Nursing Home Administrators
Suite 409
8641 Colesville Road
Silver Spring, MD 20910

American Dance Therapy Association
2000 Century Plaza
Suite 230
Columbia, MD 21044

American Dental Association
21 East Chicago Avenue
Chicago, IL 60611

American Dietetic Association
430 North Michigan Avenue
Chicago, IL 60611

American Foundation for the Blind
15 West 16th Street
New York, NY 10011
(212) 620-2000

American Geriatrics Society, Inc.
10 Columbus Circle, NW
Washington, D.C. 20006

American Health Care Association
1200 Fifteenth Street, NW
Washington, D.C. 20005

American Heart Association
7320 Greenville
Dallas, TX 75231

American Hospital Association
840 North Lake Shore Drive
Chicago, IL 60611

American Medical Association
535 Dearborn Street
Chicago, IL 60605

American Medical Technologists
710 Higgins Road
Park Ridge, IL 60068

American Nurses' Association
7320 Pershing Road
Kansas City, MO 64108

American Occupational Therapy Association
1383 Piccard Drive
Rockville, MD 20850
(301) 948-9626

American Optometric Association
7000 Chippewa Street
St. Louis, MO 63119

American Orthotic and Prosthetic Association
1440 N Street, NW
Washington, D.C. 20005

American Osteopathic Association
212 East Ohio Street
Chicago, IL 60611

American Personnel and Guidance Association
Two Skyline Place
Suite 400
5203 Leesburg Pike
Falls Church, VA 22041

American Pharmaceutical Association
2215 Constitution Avenue NW
Washington, DC 20037

American Physical Therapy Association
1111 North Fairfax Street
Alexandria, VA 22314

American Podiatric Association
20 Chevy Chase Circle, NW
Washington, D.C. 20015

American Psychological Association
Clinical Psychology Division of Adult Development and Aging
1200 7th Street, NW
Washington, D.C. 20036

American Social Health Association
1740 Broadway
New York, NY 10019

American Speech and Hearing Association
10301 Rockville Pike
Rockville, MD 20850
(301) 897-5700

Architectural and Transportation Barriers Compliance Board
Office of Human Development
U.S. Department of Health and Human Services
330 C Street, SW
Washington, D.C.
(202) 245-1591

Association of Health Facility Licensure and Certification Directors
c/o Rhode Island Department of Health
75 Davis Street
Providence, RI 02908

Gerontological Society
1835 K Street, NW
Washington, D.C. 20006

Legal Research and Services for the Elderly
1511 K Street, NW
Washington, D.C. 20005
(202) 638-4351

National Association for Spanish Speaking Elderly
3875 Wilshire Boulevard
Suite 401
Los Angeles, CA 90005
(213) 487-1922

National Association of Social Workers
Suite 600
1425 H Street, NW
Washington, D.C.

National Association of the Deaf
814 Thayer Avenue
Silver Spring, MD 20910
(301) 587-1788

National Caucus on the Black Aged
Suite 811
1730 M Street, NW
Washington, D.C. 20036

National Citizen Coalition for Nursing Home Reforms
Elma Griesal National Paralegal Institute
2000 P Street, NW
Washington, D.C. 20036

National Council of Health Care Services
Suite 402
1200 15th Street, NW
Washington, D.C. 20005

National Indian Council on Aging, Inc.
P.O. Box 2088
Albuquerque, NM 87103
(505) 766-2276

National Institute of Adult Day Care
600 Maryland Avenue, SW
West Wing 100
Washington, D.C. 20024
(202) 479-1200

Office of Handicapped Individuals
Office of Human Development Services
U.S. Department of Health and Human Services
200 Independence Avenue, SW
Washington, D.C. 20201
(202) 245-6644

Appendix A
Focus on Geriatric Care & Rehabilitation*

PREVENTION AND MANAGEMENT OF PRESSURE SORES: NEW TECHNIQUES FOR AN OLD PROBLEM

Putting the Problem in Perspective

Pressure sores have plagued caregivers and patients since the advent of medical history. We know how they are caused and how to prevent them. Yet some 3% of patients in acute care hospitals and 45% of chronically hospitalized patients develop these debilitating wounds.[1] They are potential causes of infection, suffering, and disability. Once a pressure sore develops, nursing costs can increase by up to 50%.[2] Each pressure ulcer costs between $14,000 and $25,000 to treat,[1,3,4] totaling over $2 billion per year.

Why are pressure sores so prevalent in the elderly? The answer appears obvious. Aged skin is fragile and chair-bound or bedridden geriatric patients spend large periods of time in the same position. Factor in incontinence and restraints, and the patient is at risk. But other contributing problems are sometimes overlooked, including poor nutrition, deteriorated mental status, and dehydration secondary to diuretics. Certain commercial devices, such as "pressure rings" and various foam protectors intended to prevent local pressure, ironically make matters worse. Finally, many nurses do not implement current research findings because they are unaware of new treatments, skeptical, or prohibited from initiating care on their own.[5]

*Reprinted from Focus on Geriatric Care & Rehabilitation, Vol. 1, No. 3, Aspen Publishers, Inc., © July/August 1987.

The good news is that clinicians are discarding many old misconceptions about pressure sores and developing new approaches to care. The axiom, "Where there's no pressure, there's no sore," still holds true. Preventive management centers on understanding the pathophysiology of pressure sores, defining patients at high risk,[6,7] and preventing pressure-induced ischemia.

When prevention fails, we now take a more physiologic approach to management and treat pressure sores by stage.[2,8–10] Caregivers formerly provided care by trial and error, applying sugar, lotions, heat, and a host of other substances that have no documented efficacy. Conventional wet-to-dry dressings have come under attack, because they debride granulating tissue along with necrotic areas. Current care (and the wave of the future) is the moisture vapor-permeable dressing.[11–16] These dressings mimic the body's own heating environment. They cut down sharply on time spent changing dressings and therefore reduce cost.

This article provides a practical, easily used format for preventing pressure sores in the geriatric setting and a protocol for treating them when they develop. Clinicians who understand sound physiologic principles and plan care accordingly can expect better recovery rates, reduced patient disability, and lower costs of care.

Calling Pressure Sores by Their Proper Names

Pressure sores develop when a patient at risk lies in one position for an extended period of time and cuts off blood supply to vulnerable areas. The common term *decubitus ulcer* is actually a misnomer, because it derives from the Latin word *decub* (to lie down).[17] But a large percentage of pressure sores also develop while patients are sitting. Therefore the terms *pressure sore* and *pressure ulcer* more accurately define the wound.

Prevention: Understanding and Eliminating Etiologic Factors

You'd obviously rather prevent pressure sores than treat them. It is important to predict which patients are at risk and to understand and minimize the forces that cause pressure sores. This understanding provides the basis for both prevention and management.

Predicting susceptibility

Seventy percent of pressure sores in hospitalized patients occur within two weeks of admission, making a thorough initial skin assessment essential.[1] The Norton Score (a five-point assessment of risk factors) provides a rapid means of evaluation. Evaluating the patient's physical condition, mental status, activity, mobility, and level of incontinence, it predicts susceptibility to pressure sores with a high degree of accuracy.[7] Rate your patient in each of the 5 categories on a scale of 1 to 4. A score of of 17–20 indicates that a patient is healthy, active and alert and at low risk for pressure sores. Patients scoring 14 or less are high-risk candidates and require all-out preventive efforts.

Reevaluate elderly patients frequently: pressure sore risk assessment is not a one-time measure. Any changes in one of the five risk categories changes risk status.

Ninety-six percent of pressure sores occur on the lower body, particularly over bony prominences.[17] Part of daily care for high-risk patients includes inspecting the sacral and coccygeal areas, the ischial tuberosities, and greater trochanter.[18] Also look for development of pressure areas on the elbows, shoulders, ankles, heels, and knees.

Skin folds and the groin require inspection for break-down. These areas become moist and macerated, particularly in obese or incontinent individuals.

Forces that Cause Pressure Sores

Four critical factors contribute to pressure sores. Take measures to eliminate them in all susceptible patients.

- **Pressure:** Constant skin and soft tissue pressure, particularly over bony prominences, increases interstitial pressure and venous and lymphatic obstruction. These factors lead to destruction and accumulation of metabolic waste products.

The Norton Score

Physical Condition		Mental State		Activity		Mobility		Incontinence	
Good	4	Alert	4	Ambulatory	4	Full	4	None	4
Fair	3	Apathetic	3	Walks with help	3	Slightly limited	3	Occasional	3
Poor	2	Confused	2	Chair bound	2	Very limited	2	Usually urine	2
Very bad	1	Stuporous	1	Bedridden	1	Immobile	1	Urine/fecal	1

Stage 1 ulcers may develop in debilitated patients who remain in the same position for as little as two hours.

Repositioning patients at least every two hours is essential. Turn the patient from side to side and back to front. Use small pillows to support edematous extremities, separate the knees and feet, and prop the patient on the designated side.

Chair-bound patients require weight shifts every 15–30 minutes (independently or assisted by staff). Use of an eggcrate or resilient foam cushion, an air pillow, or a gel flotation pad helps to decrease pressure but does not substitute for weight shifts.[19] Adjust the foot-rests so that the weight of the legs is partially supported by the feet and the backs of the thighs are not compressed against the seat.

- **Shearing forces** result when the caregivers elevate the head of the bed more than 30 degrees (Fowler's position) and the patient slides down. These forces also develop when the patient is sitting in a wheelchair that is not well supported. Shearing produces capillary compression, stretching of blood vessels, and compromised blood flow to the sacrum and deep fascia. When combined with direct pressure, it causes most sacral and coccygeal lesions.[2] To prevent shearing forces, do not elevate the head of the bed.

Figure 1 Pressure Points Prone to Ulceration

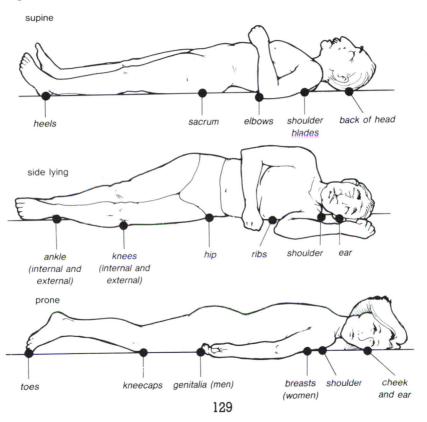

supine

heels   sacrum   elbows   shoulder blades   back of head

side lying

ankle (internal and external)   knees (internal and external)   hip   ribs   shoulder   ear

prone

toes   kneecaps   genitalia (men)   breasts (women)   shoulder   cheek and ear

Patients with respiratory difficulties or reflux esophagitis who require a high Fowler's position should have a firmly braced footboard to prevent sliding down in the bed. Sheepskins reduce shear, making them particularly important for bedridden patients.[17]

- **Friction** is produced when patients are pulled up in bed or across an examining table or when spasticity causes an extremity to rub against an adjacent surface.[2] Friction denudes the epidermis and paves the way for pressure sore development.[17]

Prevent frictional forces by lifing, rather than dragging, the patient up in bed. Two or more people should move the patient, using a drawsheet if necessary. Never pull a patient across any surface. When administering skin care, pat the skin rather than rub it (which creates friction).

- **Moisture** due to urinary or fecal incontinence increases the risk of pressure sore formation fivefold.[17] Wet skin macerates and may slough or tear.

Meticulous care is a must for incontinent patients, who are prone to pressure sores. Other important considerations include changing the linen if the patient perspires profusely and keeping clothes and bedsheets free of food particles.

Figure 2 Compression of soft tissues between the underlying surface and the bony prominence leads to the generation of a cone shaped pressure gradient with the base of the cone on the bone. *Source:* Reprinted from "The Pressure Sore: Pathophysiology and Principles of Management" by J.B. Reuler and T.B. Rooney in *Annals of Internal Medicine,* Vol. 94, pp. 661–666 with permission of American College of Physicians, © 1981.

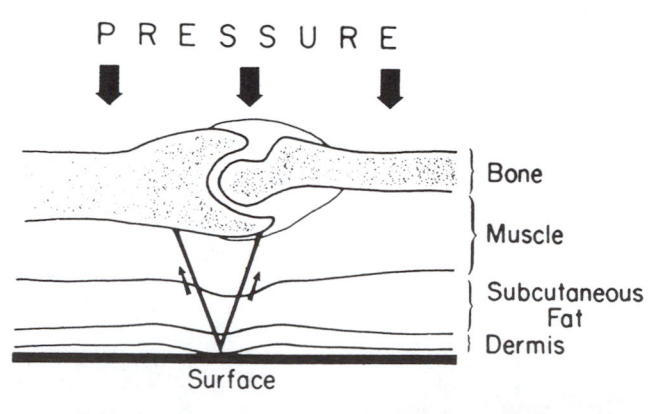

Special protective devices are useful adjuncts to frequent repositioning. The mattresses described are available as seat cushions for wheelchair-bound patients. Consider using the following devices:

- An overhead trapeze to help alert and able patients to reposition themselves.

- Sheepskin heel and elbow protectors to reduce friction.

- Knee abductor pads.

- Firm, flat wheelchair seats. Use a seatboard, if necessary, and provide appropriate padding (foam, air or water cushions, gel flotation pillows).

- ROHO air cushions, particularly suitable for incontinent patients.[19]

- Foam wedges that promote 90 degree hip flexion to keep the patient up in bed and prevent shearing.

- Foam seat cushions (should be 4 inches thick).

- Sheepskin pads, available as synthetic or genuine sheepskin. Use synthetic sheepskin when

---

Staging Pressure Sores

Look for the following signs to gauge the depth of the sore and plan treatment accordingly:

Stage 1. The cardinal sign is reddened skin that persists for more than two hours after alleviating pressure. The skin and the underlying tissue remain soft and intact.

Stage 2. Redness persists, usually accompanied by edema and induration. The outer skin layer may blister or erode.

Stage 3. An open lesion that extends to the subcutaneous tissue characterizes this stage. You may be able to see fascia at the base of the ulcer.

Stage 4. Necrosis extends through the fascia and may involve the bone, causing osteomyelitis. Eschar formation is common. It is difficult to distinguish Stage 3 from Stage 4 pressure sores prior to debridement.

---

the patient is incontinent, because its mesh backing allows urine to drain through to an incontinence pad placed beneath it.[20] Genuine sheepskin is backed with the animal's hide, which is impervious to moisture and promotes skin maceration. Either sheepskin is appropri-

Risk Factors for Pressure Sores

Elderly and neurologically impaired persons are at highest risk for pressure sores. The following factors increase risk:

Aged skin (diminished epidermal thickness, dermal collagen, and elasticity)

Diuretics (can lead to poor skin turgor)

Restricted mobility

Urinary or fecal incontinence

Impaired mental status (confusion, dementia)

Neurological impairment and its manifestations (paralysis, spasticity, decreased sensation)

Moisture and heat

Factors that impair cellular metabolism (anemia, blood dyscrasias, blood vessel fragility)

Cardiovascular disease

Edema (due to any cause)

ate to place under the feet and legs of patients with poor circulation.

- Eggcrate mattresses (polyurethane foam mattresses, about 1½ inches thick). Use at least three of these (about 4 inches total thickness). These dissipate pressure by allowing greater body surface contact with the supporting surface and can be cut to accommodate a gel flotation pad. You can also fashion wheelchair seat cushions from these.

- Gel flotation pads (a synthetic cushion filled with a synthetic substance that approximates the consistency of human fat). Place these pads under vulnerable areas (or under a pressure sore, if one has already developed). Flotation pads reduce pressure under the ischial tuberosities when the patient is sitting upright: a bed pillow is ineffective. The pads may also be placed into an opening cut in the eggcrate mattress to reduce pressure on bony prominences or pressure sores that have already developed.

- Air mattresses reduce pressure moderately but not enough to maintain blood flow to all capillaries. They may actually create pressure points in edematous or obese patients. A tight-fitting foundation sheet negates all friction-reducing properties of air mattresses, and air mattresses do not reduce shear.[20] Air pressure mattresses offer no significant advantages over foam mattresses, are more expensive, and more difficult to maintain.[21,22]

- Water mattresses provide uniform body support and may reduce pressure enough to maintain adequate capillary flow. But the waterproof covering prevents perspiration from evaporating, and even mild sweating can produce friction when the patient moves. These mattresses therefore may induce skin maceration. Some patients feel cold or actually become hypothermic on these mattresses, which have no heating system. Consider using sheepskin in combination with this mattress. Water mattresses are unsuitable for patients who weigh over 300 pounds.

The Well-Made Bed

1. Use an eggcrate mattress (polyurethane foam) over the foundation mattress to reduce pressure on all body parts. You'll need up to three of these matresses (about 4 inches thick) to achieve the desired effect. Eggcrate mattresses can also be cut to accommodate a gel flotation pad.
2. Tuck in the sheets securely, but not so tightly that they prevent the foam or gel from conforming to body contours. Keep the linen dry and wrinkle free.
3. Reduce friction by applying a thin layer of cornstarch on the foundation sheet.
4. Use Kylie sheets, if available. These have been shown to draw urine away from the patient and tend not to wrinkle as much as other sheets.
5. Use of an artificial sheepskin reduces pressure and drains urine if the patient is incontinent. Protect the foundation sheet and matress by placing a disposable incontinence pad under the sheepskin.
6. Never place plastic-backed incontinence pads directly under the patient. The plastic retains urine and increases body heat, causing skin maceration.
7. Sheepskins are impractical for patients with fecal incontinence. Instead, place a soft drawsheet over a plastic incontinence pad.
8. Use a bed cradle to prevent top sheets and blankets from resting on the patient's legs and feet.

- The Clinitron flotation system reduces pressure to the maximum degree. "Flotation" is caused by the constant motion of silicon beads in the mattress. The Clinitron system is extremely useful for patients who cannot tolerate any pressure at all or who are completely bedridden. Its two main disadvantages are its cost and the fact that the bed cannot be raised or lowered to assist transfer. (A low-position model is available, but this makes nursing care difficult.)

Avoid hammocks, because these place weight on the ischial tuberosities and sacrum.

When Prevention Fails: Principles of Treatment

Not all pressure sores are preventable, despite the best care. Malnourished, emaciated patients have neither the padding the body needs to prevent pressure sores nor the protein stores necessary to heal them. You also cannot prevent tissue breakdown in elderly or debilitated persons who

Information Alert

Myths and Misconceptions About Common Pressure Sore Remedies

Substance	Action
Hydrogen peroxide	Causes debris to surface; has some bactericidal effect. Does not promote healing; destroys all new epithelial cells. Never instill into closed body cavity: released gas cannot escape. Rinse well.
Betadine solution	Bactericidal; does not promote healing. Toxic when absorbed; rinse well.
PhisoHex	Destroys new epithelial cells; may encourage growth of *Pseudomonas*.
Silver nitrate	Does not promote healing or prevent infection. Very caustic.
Sugar	No proven therapeutic value.
Antacids	No proven therapeutic value.
Reston	Creates added pressure when patient lies on this substance. Acceptable for use between fingers and toes or around anal area.

fall prior to admission and lie on the affected area. Patients with spasticity due to neurologic impairment are prime candidates for pressure sores unless the problem is corrected. With all stages of pressure sores, the most important factor is to keep pressure off the wound. No treatment can be effective unless pressure is relieved.

Avoid folk remedies

Research over the last few years has demonstrated that certain time-honored methods of treating pressure sores may do more harm than good. Caregivers have applied everything from table sugar to maggots; most of these methods have no proven clinical benefit. Wet-to-dry dressings, while appropriate for debridement, should be used with caution. These dressings must be changed several times daily, and removal of the old packing often tears away new granulating tissue. They can also cause the patient considerable pain during removal if the tissue is healing.

Basic Principles of Dressings and Wound Care

1. Wash your hands thoroughly before and after the procedure.
2. Gather all necessary equipment at the bedside. Be certain that saline intended for irrigation has been warmed to body temperature.
3. Explain the procedure to the patient. (Confused or demented patients may require reminding and explanation prior to each dressing change.) If the dressing change is painful, premedicate the patient as ordered.
4. Wear sterile gloves to remove the old dressing. Pull the tape toward the wound to avoid strain on the site. Use a tape remover if the tape does not come off easily.
5. Note any signs of infection (increased reddening, foul odor, increased drainage or change in color, or pus). If the wound has been packed with gauze, moisten it with warm saline before removing it.
6. Change to new sterile gloves before applying the new dressing.
7. Avoid using adhesive tape on the elderly patient's skin. Paper tape or Montgomery straps reduce the need for adhesive tape.

Moisture vapor-permeable dressings promote healing

A warm, moist environment, coupled with relief of pressure, is the ideal way to manage noninfected pressure sores. Semipermeable hydrocolloid dressings, the current state of the art, encourage debridement and granulation[11,12,14] and often heal ulcers that fail to respond to conventional therapy.[16] These are adhesive dressings that are permeable to air but not to moisture. They interact physically with the wound fluid and promote healing by speeding the rate of epithelial migration.[20] Other advantages include less pain for the patient (because the dressing covers exposed nerve endings) and decreased frequency of dressing change. Unless the dressing leaks, it may be left in place for 7–10 days, which cuts down considerably on nursing time and costs.

Dressings commonly in use include DuoDERM, Op-Site, and Tegaderm. Tegaderm and Op-Site are transparent, but DuoDERM is not. However, DuoDERM seems to cause less skin trauma when removed. Before applying these dressings, be certain that the wound is not infected, because the warm, moist environment will stimulate bacterial proliferation.

Stage 1

Management consists of keeping body weight off the reddened area. Do not massage the reddened area, because this causes further tissue damage. With proper care, healing should occur within several days. A check on other body parts is essential. Moving the patient off one area may place another area at higher risk for pressure sore development.

Evaluate the patient and institute protective measures according to individual needs. Patients who develop Stage 1 pressure sores require (at minimum) eggcrate mattresses, sheepskin protectors of the bony prominences, frequent turning, meticulous skin care, and nutritional evaluation.

Stage 2

Do not apply lotions, ointments, or drying soaps on broken skin. Wash the pressure sore with half-strength Betadine, making certain to rinse well with normal saline, and dry the surrounding area thoroughly. Apply the hydrocolloid dressing over the wound site, leaving a 1- to 1½-inch margin. Unless the dressing loosens or drainage appears, you can leave the dressing undisturbed for 7–10 days. Stage 1 protocols then apply. If the patient develops a fever, remove the dressing and consider culturing the wound.

For draining of infected Stage 2 pressure sores, place the patient in a whirlpool bath to cleanse the site. Then apply Domeboro's solution, an antiseptic used exclusively for draining Stage 2 wounds. This is supplied as a powder that must be dissolved in water to provide the desired strength. Apply the solution as soaks three to four times daily for 30 minutes. Apply a dry sterile dressing after the soaks or leave the area open to air if it is not draining excessively.

Once the infection resolves, continue treatment with a moisture vapor-permeable dressing as described above. Use of antacids,[23] sugar, creams, or pastes has no place in the management of open wounds. Exposing the area to a heat lamp only worsens matters, because this dries and cracks the skin.

Stage 3

These pressure sores are sometimes infected and often contain necrotic tissue. The sore is sometimes covered with eschar (a hard, blackened formation not to be confused with a healthy scab found on cuts and abrasions). This must be debrided. These pressure sores may be either painful or devoid of sensation secondary to destruction of nerve endings.

If the wound is infected and draining, begin irrigation with quarter-strength hydrogen peroxide. Never irrigate forcefully, and do not use this solution in a closed body cavity (for example, a parianal pressure sore with suspected rectal involvement). Hydrogen peroxide decomposes into oxygen and water when exposed to blood, and the liberated gases cannot escape. Discontinue use as soon as the wound is clean.

Necrotic wounds or those with eschar require surgical, mechanical, or chemical debridement.

The method of debridement depends on the extent of the damage. Most facilities use wet-to-dry saline dressings for mechanical debridement. These should only be used as long as necrotic tissue is present, because removal of the packing tears away granulating tissue as well. To apply a wet-to-dry dressing:

- Assemble sterile gloves, warmed saline, sterile bowls, towels, Kling dressing, and dry gauze pads.

- After donning sterile gloves, soak the Kling dressing in normal saline. Moisten the old packing with saline and remove.

- Note the appearance of the wound and the color and consistency of material on the old dressing. Be sure no old gauze pads are left in the wound.

- After changing sterile gloves, irrigate the wound, if necessary. Be certain to flush out all irrigant.

- Wring out the Kling dressing and use it to pack the wound. The gauze should be moist but not moist enough to leak. Cut off excess gauze.

- Cover the site with an abdominal dressing pad and secure with Montgomery straps.

- Change the dressing every 4 to 6 hours.

- Discontinue these dressings as soon as all necrotic tissue has been removed.

Pressure sores that are covered with eschar require whirlpool or surgical or enzymatic debridement. A number of enzymatic products are available (for example, Santyl, Elase, Travase). To cleanse a wound with an enzymatic product:

- Clean the wound first with peroxide, then saline. Don't use solutions containing heavy metal ions, such as Betadine, PhisoHex, or Burrow's solution. These solutions negate the enzyme's activity.

- Protect the wound edges with karaya, which spares viable tissue from enzymatic destruction.[24]

Basic Skin Care for Elderly and/or Debilitated Patients

1. Soap dries the skin and may do more harm than good. Most elderly patients do not require a full bath every day and do well with a tube bath or shower once or twice weekly. Offer sponge baths in between full baths or showers.

2. After washing, do not rub the skin dry. Pat it with an absorbent towel.

3. Skin areas that are wet or stool-covered should be immediately and throughly cleaned and patted dry.

4. Lotions are appropriate for use on unbroken skin only.

5. Check all pressure points and bony prominences daily and document these in the chart. Signs of skin breakdown occur here first.

6. Foot care is important in all patients, but particularly those who are diabetic or who have neurocirculatory impairment. Have patients soak their feet in warm water with an emollient, such as a bath oil. Inspect for bunions, blisters, ingrown toenails, signs of inflammation, and breaks in the skin. Pressure sores usually develop first over the heels and bony prominences of the ankle.

7. All patients at risk for pressure sores require heel and elbow protectors.

8. Patients with paralysis or beginning contractures require evaluation by a physical therapist. Apply passive range of motion and splint the hand or foot in a position of function (using lamb's wool or Reston between the digits).

- Spread a thin layer of the enzyme preparation onto a dry gauze pad, then pack the ulcer with the gauze. Cover the packing with plastic wrap, which will keep the packing moist.

- Change the dressing every 24 hours until the ulcer is debrided.

- Monitor the patient for general condition changes and nutritional improvement.

Hydrophilic beads, such as Debrisan, absorb fluid and inhibit exudate that prevents healing. These beads do not digest necrotic tissue, debride eschar, or cleanse nonsecreting pressure sores. They do promote a moist, healing environment without sealing off the wound for several days (as with the hydrocolloid dressings) and risking an incubating infection. To use Debrisan:[24]

- Assemble Debrisan, sterile saline, irrigating equipment, sterile containers, gauze pads, benzoin, and tape.

- Irrigate or cleanse the ulcer, rinse with saline, and dry the outer edges.

- Pour the Debrisan beads into the ulcer, creating a $1/4$- to $1/8$-inch deep layer. Place a sterile gauze dressing over the ulcer and secure with paper tape. Cover the gauze with plastic wrap, leaving room for the beads to expand as they absorb fluid.

- When the ulcer is difficult to reach, Debrisan may also be made into a paste by mixing 4:1 with glycerine. The edges of the pressure sore are protected with karaya and the paste applied with a sterile applicator. Cover with gauze.

- Change the dressings once or twice daily, or more if the sore is draining profusely.

Stage 4

In addition to measures used for Stage 3 ulcers, these are usually managed surgically.[17] Wound care is essentially the same as Stage 3, and observation of the patient for associated sepsis is paramount.

Proper Nutrition is Essential

Malnourished patients have a poor rate of recovery from pressure sores, regardless of what is done to the wound. Caregivers should keep a sharp watch on the patient's calorie count and quality of food consumed. Elderly people are often placed on a pureed diet with little or no rationale. These diets tend to be very unpalatable, leading to decreased intake and increased risk of malnourishment. Important dietary measures include the following:

- If the patient has dentures, be sure they fit well.

- Allow a mechanical soft diet, if possible. This diet offers improved texture, taste, and smell over pureed food. Most patients can eat this food (even without dentures) if the meat is properly prepared.

- Assist patients with feeding when necessary.

- Don't give the patient dessert (usually empty calories) until the main meal is eaten.

- Offer high-protein snacks.

- Liquid high-calorie supplements can be made more palatable by blenderizing them with ice. Before offering this "milkshake," give the patient a small drink of lemonade or apple juice. This will help avoid the thickened secretions these supplements often produce.

PRACTICAL TIPS ON PREVENTING AND MANAGING PRESSURE SORES

- Evaluate the risk status on all patients, using the Norton Score.

- Check and recheck skin condition of high-risk patients every week.

- Implement prevention and/or treatment protocol immediately and consistently.

- Use a flow sheet for positioning patients. Note the time the patient was repositioned, the new position, and any changes in skin integrity. Bedridden patients require turning at least every two hours. Chair-bound patients should change position every 15–30 minutes. Wheelchair "pushups" are helpful if the patient has sufficient arm strength.

- Keep patients out of bed as much as possible.

- Educate patients, if feasible. Emphasize the importance of moving themselves, not sliding down in the bed (which causes shear), and remaining out of bed.

- Use assistive devices to reduce pressure and friction. All patients at risk require at least sheepskin, eggcrate mattresses, heel and elbow protectors, and wheelchair cushions.

- Provide thorough and prompt incontinence care when necessary. Wash the skin and pat it dry. Do not rub.

- Do not allow any elderly patient to sit on the bedpan for more than a few minutes, because pressure sores may develop due to constriction of blood vessels.

- Do not use folk remedies on pressure sores if they develop. The use of heat or drying agents makes matters worse.

- No treatment works unless the patient is kept off the affected site.

- Be certain that the patient is eating at least three high-protein meals daily. Keep a calorie count if there is any doubt. Provide high-protein snacks between meals, and avoid junk foods.

REFERENCES

1. Kenedi RM, Cowden MJ, Scales JT, eds. Bedsore biomechanics. Baltimore: University Park Press, 1976.

2. DeLisa JA, Mikulic MA. Pressure ulcers: what to do if preventive management fails. Postgrad Med 1985; 77:209–220.

3. Vistnes LM. Pressure sores: etiology and treatment. Washington, DC: National Merit Proposal, Veterans Administration Office, 1979.

4. Sather MR, Weber CE Jr., George J. Pressure sores and the spinal cord injury patient. Drug Intell Clin Pharm 1977; 11:154–169.

5. Gould D. Pressure sore prevention and treatment: an example of nurses' failure to implement research findings. J Adv Nurs 1986; 11:389–394.

6. Lincoln R, Roberts R, Maddox A, et al. Use of the Norton pressure sore risk assessment scoring system with elderly patients in acute care. J Enterostom Ther 1986; 13:132–138.

7. Goldstone LA, Goldstone J. The Nortn score: an early warning of pressure sores? J Adv Nurs 1982; 7:419–426.

8. Cassel BL. Treating pressure sores stage by stage. RN 1986; 49:36–41.

9. Pictorial: staging care for pressure sores. Am J Nurs 1984; 84:999–1003.

10. Smith DB, ed. Toward a physiologic approach to the topical management of open wounds. J Enterostom Ther 1983; 10:101–107.

11. Sebern MD. Pressure ulcer management in home care: efficacy and cost-effectiveness of moisture vapor permeable dressing. Arch Phys Med Rehabil 1986; 67:726–729.

12. Fellin R. Managing decubitus ulcers. Cost savings by substituting hydrocolloid for gauze dressings. Nurs Manage 1984; 15:29–30.

13. Lingner C, Rolstad BS, Wethrill K, Danielson S. Clinical trial of a moisture vapor-permeable dressing on superficial pressure sores. J Enterostom Ther 1984; 11:147–149.
14. Tudhope M. Management of pressure ulcers with a hydrocolloid occlusive dressing: results in twenty-three patients. J Enterostom Ther 1984; 11:102–105.
15. Fowler E, Goupil DL. Comparison of the wet-to-dry dressing and a copolymer starch in the management of debrided pressure sores. J Enterostom Ther 1984; 11:22–25.
16. Yarnosky GM, Kramer E, King R, et al. Pressure sore management: efficacy of a moisture-reactive occlusive dressing. Arch Phys Med Rehabil 1984: 65:597–600.
17. Reuler JB, Cooney TB. The pressure sore: pathology and principles of management. Ann Intern Med 1981; 94:661–666.
18. Ek AC, Boman G. A descriptive study of pressure sores: the prevalence of pressure sores and the characteristics of patients. J Adv Nurs 1982; 7:51–57.
19. Krouskop TA, Noble PC, Garber SL, Spencer WA. The effectiveness of preventive management in reducing the occurrence of pressure sores. J Rehabil R&D 1983; 20:74–83.
20. Waldo L. 5 famous fallacies about pressure sores. Nursing 84 1984; 14:34–41.
21. Daechsel D, Conine T. Special mattresses: effectiveness in preventing decubitus ulcers in chronic neurologic patients. Arch Phys Med Rehabil 1985; 66:246–248.
22. Whitney JD, Fellows BJ, Larson E. Do mattresses make a difference? J Gerontol Nurs 1984; 10:20–25.
23. Becker L, Goodemonte C. Treating pressure sores with or without antacid. Am J Nurs 1984; 84:351–352.
24. Arnell I. Treating decubitus ulcers: two methods that work. Nursing 1983; 13:50–55.

BOOKS AND ARTICLES
for Staff Inservice or Family or Patient Education

Parrish LC, Witowski JA, Crissey JT. *The Decubitus Ulcer.* New York: Year Book Medical Publishers, 1985.
Pictorial: staging care for pressure sores. *American Journal of Nursing,* 1984; 84:999–1003.
Waldo, L. 5 famous fallacies about pressure sores. *Nursing 84* 1984; 14:34–41.

Appendix B
Self Balance Hints for Older Persons*

NO ONE WANTS TO GO TO THE HOSPITAL

One way to avoid the need for hospital stays is to take care to prevent falls, since falls are one of the main reasons that older persons are admitted to hospitals or to long-stay institutions.

Geriatric researchers agree that about 33% of people over the age of 65 have one or more falls in a year resulting in almost 10,000 deaths. Injuries from falls are the sixth leading cause of death in people over the age of 75. Of the 200,000 people who sustain a fracture of the hip each year from falls, 84% are over the age of 65 and are hospitalized an average of 21 days.

These accidents, many of which are preventable, take a devastating toll on older persons. Victims of falls may suffer life-threatening complications. Many also develop anxiety about future falls and this interferes with their continued independence. Fear of falls often results in limitation of activity, dependence and unhappiness. In the saddest of circumstances, older people are prevented from living at home because of potentially treatable imbalance problems.

My many years of clinical experience with older persons have borne out time and time again that if older persons took care of their bodies by stretching and strengthening their muscles, physical therapists would not see so many clients with fractured hips and balance problems.

Several ingredients make a person more at risk for falls and balance problems. Some of the major ingredients are posture, blood regulation, brain input, strength, flexibility and the environment. De-

*Reprinted from *Self Balance Hints for Older Persons* by C.B. Lewis, Aspen Publishers, Inc., © 1987.

veloping flexibility is one way of keeping fit and avoiding balance problems. Developing strength in muscle groups is a second line of defense.

Listed in this booklet are simple stretching and strengthening exercises designed specifically for an older person. These exercises will promote strength, flexibility, and coordination. In addition, I discuss ways of improving one's posture. The muscles of the leg and the thigh are areas of focus for improved posture. I also emphasize strengthening of muscles to improve the stability of the hip and lower back area.

This booklet will help you to judge how flexible, strong and well-balanced you are now. On the next page, you will find a self-balance test that you can use to assess your degree of risk for falls. This test will help you to decide whether you need to improve your flexibility, work on your strength, or simply maintain the current levels of activity and exercise that you have already achieved.

A word of *caution*—if you have any existing medical problems, do not start these exercises; if any of the exercises that are suggested in this book produce pain, do not continue with them. Consult your physical therapist or physician.

SELF BALANCE TEST

Posture

The figure below on the left illustrates good posture. Good posture ensures good body alignment

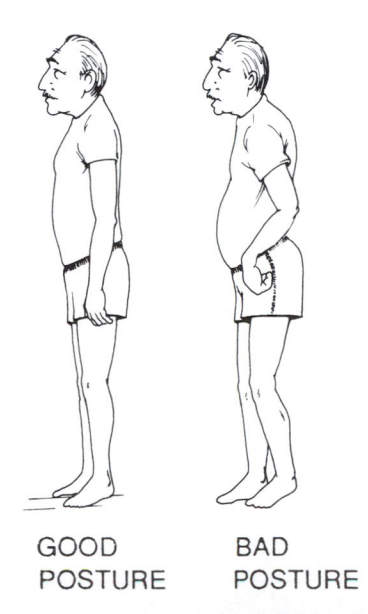

GOOD   BAD
POSTURE   POSTURE

and good balance. The righthand figure is an example of poorer posture. Poor posture can throw off the balance mechanism inherent in the body.

To Check If This Is a Problem—Have a friend look at your posture. If it is very poor, it may be necessary for you to consult a physical therapist. If it is only slightly out of alignment, you may want to try the exercises in the next section.

Blood Flow

Sometimes the heart is unable to get blood to the brain as quickly as it is needed.

To Check if This is a Problem—lie down and sit up quickly; have a friend watching for your own safety. If you feel lightheaded or dizzy, this is a sign that you may have some difficulty in this area. If the problem seems severe, consult your physician. If mild, make a commitment to yourself: Every time you change body positions (from lying to sitting or from sitting to standing) stay still and breathe deeply for 1 or 2 minutes before walking or moving actively. This will allow time for a steady flow of blood to reach your brain.

Blood flow can also be stopped or slowed temporarily by moving your head in certain ways.

To Check if This is a Problem—sit in a chair and have a friend observe your eyes. Tilt your head back as far as you can and look over one shoulder. Hold that position for a slow 10 seconds. Repeat this movement in the other direction. Note eye movement, dizziness, or nausea. If you experience any of the above symptoms, you *must* avoid these types of positions and you should consult a health professional.

Nerve Input

If we stop moving our necks because of jobs or out of habit, the brain will get less information on our neck and body positions.

To Check if This is a Problem—notice whether you turn your whole body rather than just your head when you look around. If you do tend to turn your body, you may need more stimulation to the nerve endings in your neck. One way to get this stimulation is to gently rock your head back and forth for 1 or 2 minutes before rising from bed in the morning and before falling asleep at night. This should be done every day; keep in mind, however, that you will not see the effects of better balance for several months.

Strength

You need strong muscles to propel you through any of your daily activities, such as standing, walking, turning, bending. When muscles are weak, ordinary activities can become disjointed, or difficult to perform. Weakness in your legs can be a very important factor in loss of balance. If you are very weak in your hips or thighs you should see a physical therapist who can design an exercise program to improve your muscle strength. The foot and lower leg strength is often the key culprit and can be easily assessed and treated.

To Check if This is a Problem—try to hop on one foot; if you cannot do this, there may be muscle weakness. To strengthen these muscles simply rise up and down on your toes. Start with 10, progress by increments of 10 a week until you reach 100. (*See also* Exercise 5 in the next section, but note

that more repetitions are used here because muscle strengthening is targeted specifically.)

Flexibility

Flexibility is the ability to move a muscle and joint through a motion easily without significant

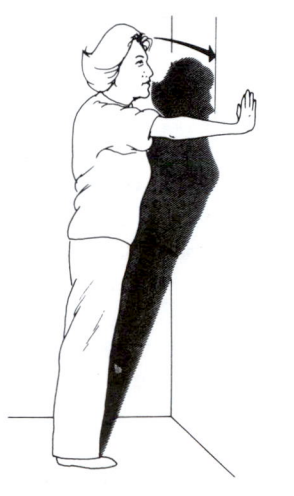

HEEL TIGHTNESS
POSITION

stress or strain on muscle or bone. Flexibility, like strength, is very important for good balance. If your muscles are very tight, consult a physical therapist. Again, legs and feet are often overlooked.

To Check if This is a Problem—stand as shown in the picture on p. 148.

If your back heel does not touch the floor as you move toward the wall, muscle tightness is indicated. As you lean into the wall, try holding the forward position for 60 seconds. Keep trying the movement described here—it is a great exercise to stretch these muscles. (It should be done *after* the exercise noted above.) This exercise is especially helpful if you always seem to catch your toe when walking.

Another tight area is the hip region. Stand in front of a mirror and try to make a circle with your hips without moving your shoulders. Look in the mirror to see whether your shoulders move when you move your hips. If so, you need to work on this area. Slowly practice these hip circles in front of a mirror without moving your shoulders. Do this 10 times in each direction.

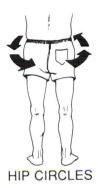

HIP CIRCLES

BALANCE EXERCISES

Here are 10 easy exercises that you can do daily to help improve flexibility and strength and thereby improve your balance. A few of these exercises were already described above. Another word of *caution:* As with any exercise, begin slowly, don't strain, and be patient. You probably won't see results for several weeks.

1 CHIN TUCKS

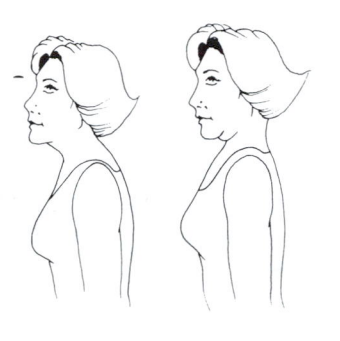

2 SHOULDERS BACK

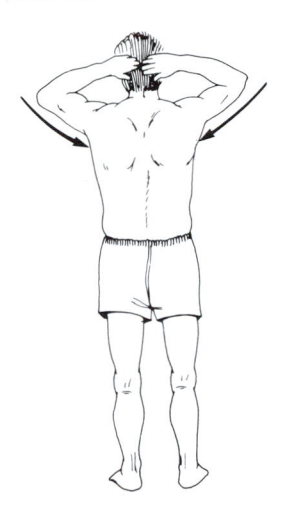

Stand as erect as you can with your neck drawn back and chin tucked in, not up. Hold head correctly; do not tilt chin. Pull neck back in line with your spine keeping chin horizontal. See picture above. Hold this position for 10 seconds, relax, breathe, and repeat 3 times.

Pull your shoulders back as if you had a piece of elastic pulling your shoulder blades together in the back. Hold that for 10 seconds and relax. Repeat three times, relaxing and breathing and holding the position for 10 seconds each time.

3 SHOULDER SHRUGS

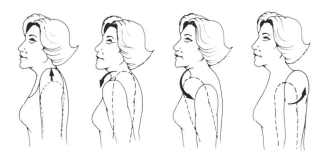

Bring your shoulders around in big circles, three times clockwise and three times counterclockwise.

4 HEAD ROCKS

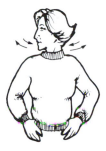

While lying down, gently rock your head from side to side 10 times.

5 TOE UPS

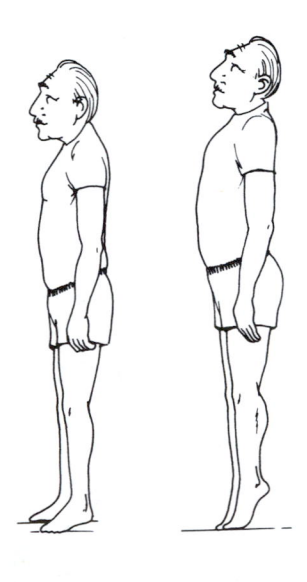

6 LEG LIFTS

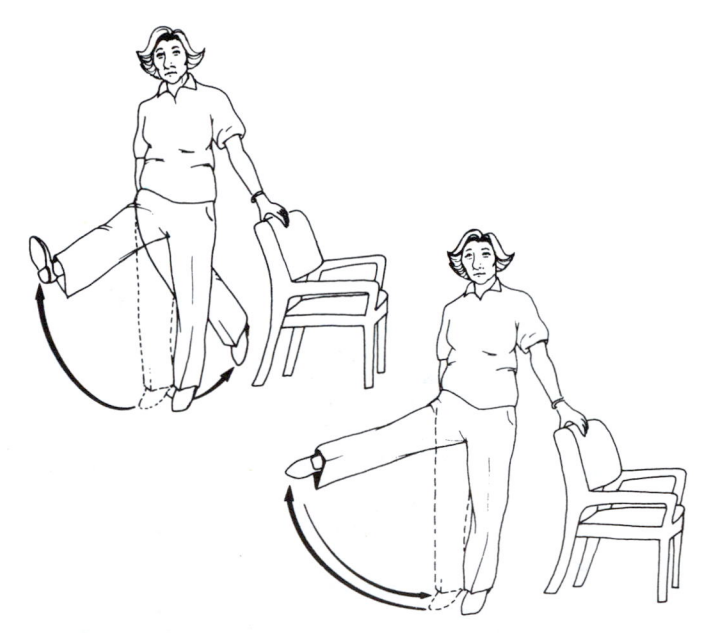

Go up on your toes as high as you can, come back down. Do this 10 times, increasing each week 5 times until you build up to 50.

Stand up and gently swing your leg back and forth 10 times; then out to the side and back 10 times.

7 QUAD SETS

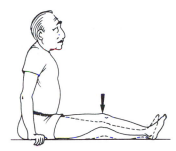

Tighten the muscles on top of the thigh *as tightly as possible* and hold. Pull 10 seconds, trying every second to pull even tighter. Relax 10 seconds.

8 RUNNER'S STRETCH

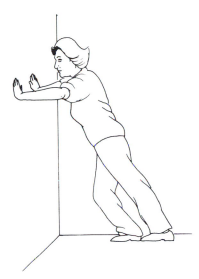

Standing with one foot behind the other, lunge forward bending front knee to stretch calf muscles in the back leg. Keep both heels flat. Hold for 10 seconds. Repeat with the other leg.

9 HIP CIRCLES

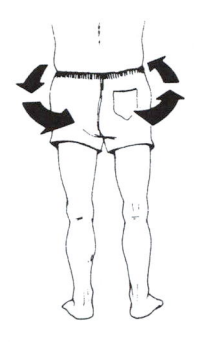

Stand in front of a mirror and make a big circle with your hip as if there were a clock around your feet. Trying not to move your shoulders, circle with your hips to one, two, three, four, etc. o'clock positions until you have made a full circle in a clockwise direction; then repeat the movement in a counterclockwise direction. Repeat 10 times in each direction.

10 GLUTEAL SETS

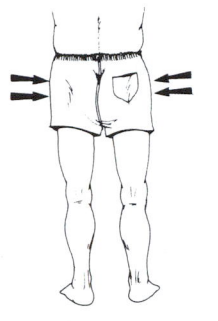

Pinch your buttocks together; hold 5 seconds, then relax. Repeat 10 times.

Appendix C
Drug Effects and Rehabilitation of the Elderly*

Table C-1. Tricyclic and Tricyclic-like Antidepressants

Generic Name	Brand Name
Amitriptyline	Elavil, Endep
Amoxapine	Asendin
Desipramine	Norpramin, Pertofrane
Doxepin	Adapin, Sinequan
Imipramine	Janimine, SK-Pramine, Tofranil
Maprotiline	Ludiomil
Nortriptyline	Avantyl, Pamelor
Protriptyline	Vivactil
Trazodone	Desyrel
Trimipramine	Surmontil

Table C-2. Selected Antipsychotic Drugs and Their Relative Incidence of Common Side Effects

Generic Name	Brand Name	Postural Hypotension	Parkinsonism	Sedation
Chlorpromazine	Thorazine	High	Moderate	High
Fluphenazine	Prolixin, Permitil	Minimal	High	Minimal
Haloperidol	Haldol	Minimal	High	Minimal
Loxapine	Loxitane	Minimal	High	Moderate
Mesoridazine	Serentil	Moderate	Minimal	High
Molindone	Moban	Minimal	High	Moderate
Perphenazine	Trilafon	Minimal	High	Minimal
Thioridazine	Mellaril	Moderate	Minimal	High
Trifluoperazine	Stelazine	Minimal	High	Minimal
Thiothixene	Navane	Minimal	High	Minimal

*Reprinted from *Topics in Geriatric Rehabilitation,* Vol. 2, No. 3, pp. 77–81, Aspen Publishers, Inc., © April 1987.

Table C-3. Commonly Used Antihypertensive Drugs and Their Relative Propensity for Causing Postural Hypotension

Generic Name	Brand Name	Postural Hypotension
Beta blockers	see Table C-6	Rare
Captopril*	Capoten	Rare
Clonidine	Catapres	Occasional
Diuretics	see Table C-4	Occasional
Enalapril*	Vasotec	Rare
Guanabenz	Wytensin	Occasional
Guanadrel	Hylorel	Common
Guanethidine	Ismelin	Common
Hydralazine	Apresoline	Rare
Labetalol	Trandate Normodyne	Occasional
Methyldopa	Aldomet	Occasional
Minoxidil	Loniten	Occasional
Prazosin†	Minipress	Occasional
Reserpine	(numerous)	Rare

*Pretreatment with a diuretic may greatly exhance the risk of postural hypotension.
† Severe postural hypotension has been noted with the initiation of therapy or with rapid and large increments in dose.

Table C-4. Diuretics That Can Cause Significant Volume Depletion and Hypokalemia

Generic Name	Brand Name
Bendroflumethiazide	Naturetin
Benzthiazide	ExNa
Bumetanide	Bumex
Chlorthalidone	Hygroton
Chlorothiazide	Diuril
Cyclothiazide	Anhydron
Ethacrynic acid	Edecrin
Furosemide	Lasix
Hydrochlorothiazide	Hyhdro-Diuril, Esidrex, Oretic
Hydroflumethiazide	Saluron
Methylclothiazide	Enduron
Metolazone	Zaroxolyn
Polythiazide	Renese
Quinethazone	Hydromox
Trichlormethiazide	Naqua

Table C-5. Nitrates

Generic Name	Brand Name
Erythrityl tetranitrate*	Cardilate
Isosorbide dinitrate*	Isordil, Sorbitrate
Nitroglycerin*†	Numerous
Pentaerythritol tetranitrate	Peritrate, Duotrate

*Also available in sublingual form.
† Also available as an ointment, spray, and transdermal patch.

Table C-6. Beta-Blocking Drugs

Generic Name	Brand Name
Acebutolol	Sectral
Atenolol	Tenormin
Metroprolol	Lopressor
Nadolol	Corgard
Pindolol	Visken
Propranolol	Inderal
Timolol	Blocadren

Table C-7. Narcotic Analgesics

Generic Name	Brand Name
Codeine*	Numerous
Hydrocodone	Hycodan
Hydromorphone	Dilaudid
Meperidine	Demerol
Methadone	Dolophine
Morphine	Numerous
Oxycodone*	Numerous
Oxymorphone	Numorphan
Pentazocine	Talwin

*Often marketed in combination with additional drugs.

Table C-8. Vasodilating Drugs

Generic Name	Brand Name
Cyclandelate	Cyclospasmol
Ergoloid mesylates	Hydergine
Ethaverine	Ethaquin, Ethatab, Laverin
Isoxsuprine	Vasodilan
Nicotinic acid	Nicobid
Nicotinyl alcohol	Roniacol
Nylidrin	Arlidin
Papaverine	Pavabid, Cerespan

Table C-9. Selected Drugs Associated with Peripheral Neuropathies

Generic Name	Brand Name
Alcohol	Numerous
Chlorambucil	Leukeran
Chloramphenicol	Chloromycetin
Cisplatin	Platinol
Dapsone	Avlosulfon
Disulfiram	Antabuse
Ethambutol	Myambutol
Gold salts	Numerous
Hydralazine	Apresoline
Isoniazid	Numerous
Metronidazole	Flagyl
Nitrofurantoin	Numerous
Penicillamine	Cuprimine, Depen
Phenytoin	Dilantin
Procarbazine	Matulane
Vincristine	Oncovin
Vinblastine	Velban

Table C-10. Selected Drugs Associated with Myopathies

Generic Name	Brand Name
Alcohol	Numerous
Chloroquine	Numerous
Clofibrate	Atromid-S
Corticosteroids	Numerous
Drug-induced hypokalemia*	Numerous
Lithium	Numerous
Penicillamine	Cuprimine, Depen
Procainamide	Pronestyl
Vincristine	Oncovin

*Primarily seen with diuretics and laxative abuse.

Table C-11. Benzodiazepines

Generic Name	Brand Name
Alprazolam	Xanax
Chlordiazepoxide	Librium
Clorazepate	Tranxene
Diazepam	Valium
Flurazepam	Dalmane
Halazepam	Paxipam
Lorazepam	Ativan
Oxazepam	Serax
Prazepam	Centrax
Quazepam	Dormalin
Triazolam	Halcion

Table C-12. Selected Drugs Associated with Depressive Reactions in the Elderly

Generic Name	Brand Name
Acetazolamide	Diamox
Alcohol	Numerous
Amantadine	Symmetrel
Antipsychotic agents	See Table C-2
Barbiturates	Numerous
Benzodiazepines	See Table C-11
Benztropine	Cogentin
Beta blockers	See Table C-6
Bromocriptine	Parlodel
Cimetidine	Tagamet
Clonidine	Catapres
Ethambutol	Myambutol
Guanabenz	Wytensin
Indomethacin	Indocin
Isoniazid	Numerous
Levodopa	Numerous
Levodopa-carbidopa	Sinemet
Methazolamide	Neptazane
Methyldopa	Aldomet
Naproxen	Naprosyn
Prazosin	Minipres
Prednisone	Numerous
Reserpine	Numerous

Table C-13. Drugs Associated with Confusional Reactions in the Elderly

Generic Name	Brand Name
Amatadine	Symmetrel
Aminophylline	Numerous
Antipsychotic agents	See Table C-2
Barbiturates	Numerous
Benzodiazepines	See Table C-11
Benztropine	Cogentin
Beta blockers	See Table C-6
Biperiden	Akineton
Bromocriptine	Parlodel
Cimetidine	Tagamet
Codeine	Numerous
Digitoxin	Crystodigin
Digoxin	Lanoxin
Indomethacin	Indocin
Isoniazid	Numerous
Levodopa	Numerous
Levodopa-carbidopa	Sinemet
Lithium	Numerous
Meperidine	Demerol
Methyldopa	Aldomet
Pentazocine	Talwin
Procyclidine	Kemadrin
Propoxyphene	Darvon
Theophylline	Numerous
Tricyclic antidepressants	See Table C-1
Trihexyphenidyl	Artane

Table C-14. Drugs Associated with Withdrawal Reactions of Which Depression or Confusion May Be an Important Component

Generic Name	Brand Name
Alcohol	Numerous
Amphetamine	Numerous
Anticholinergic agents*	Artane, Cogetin
Antipsychotic agents	See Table C-2
Baclofen	Lioresal
Barbiturates	Numerous
Benzodiazepines	See Table C-11
Clonidine	Catapres
Methylphenidate	Ritalin
Narcotic analgesics	See Table C-7
Phenytoin	Dilantin
Tricyclic antidepressants	See Table C-1

*This effect is limited to agents that partition into the brain.

Table C-15. Drugs That Can Aggravate Parkinsonism or Block the Beneficial Effects of Antiparkinson Drugs

Generic Name	Brand Name
Amoxapine	Asendin
Antipsychotic drugs	See Table C-2
Benzodiazepines*	See Table C-11
Methionine	Pedameth
Methyldopa	Aldomet
Metoclopramide	Reglan
Papaverine	Cerespan, Pavabid
Pyridoxine†	Various vitamin preparations
Reserpine	Numerous

*Further evidence for this potential adverse effect is needed.
† This potential adverse drug-drug interaction is seen only with levodopa and not in the combination preparation of levodopa-carbidopa (Sinemet).

Table C-16. Drugs That May Cause Dizziness and Vertigo by a Toxic Effect on the Vestibular System

Generic Name	Brand Name
Amikacin	Amikin
Fenoprofen	Nalfon
Gentamicin	Garamycin
Ibuprofen	Motrin
Indomethacin	Indocin
Meclofenamate	Meclomen
Naproxen	Naprosyn
Oxyphenbutazone	Tandearil, Oxalid
Phenylbutazone	Butazolidin, Azolid
Quinidine	Quinaglute, Quinidex, Quindra
Streptomycin	Numerous
Sulindac	Clinoril
Tobramycin	Nebcin
Tolmetin	Tolectin

Table C-17. Other Drugs That May Cause Dizziness or Vertigo*

Generic Name	Brand Name
Acetazolamide	Diamox
Alcohol	Numerous
Barbiturates	Numerous
Benzodiazepines	See Table C-11
Beta-adrenergic blockers	See Table C-6
Cimetidine	Tagamet
Diphenhydramine	Benadryl
Hypoglycemic agents†	Numerous
Isoniazid	Numerous
Meprobamate	Equanil, Miltown
Metronidazole	Flagyl
Mexiletine	Mexitil
Minocycline	Minocin
Nalidixic acid	NegGram
Narcotic analgesics	See Table C-7
Nifedipine	Procardia
Nitrofurantoin	Macrodantin, Furantoin, Cyantin
Oxolinic acid	Utibid
Pentoxifylline	Trental
Phenytoin	Dilantin
Primidone	Mysoline
Tocainide	Tonocard
Tricyclic antidepressants	See Table C-1
Verapamil	Isoptin, Calan

*Antihypertensive drugs or other drugs capable of causing postural hypotension can precipitate these symptoms.
† Symptoms related to excessive reduction of blood glucose.

Table C-18. Drugs Associated with Ataxic Reactions

Generic Name	Brand Name
Alcohol	Numerous
Barbiturates	Numerous
Benzodiazepines	See Table C-11
Carbamazepine	Tegretol
Levodopa-carbidopa	Sinemet
Levodopa	Dopar, Laradopa, Parda
Indomethacin	Indocin
Lithium	Eskalith, Lithane
Minocycline	Minocin
Nitrofurantoin	Macrodantin, Furadantin, Cyantin
Phenytoin	Dilantin
Valproic acid	Depakene

Table C-19.   Selected Drugs with Potent
Anticholinergic Action

Generic Name	Brand Name
Amitriptyline	Elavil, Endep
Amoxapine	Asendin
Benztropine	Cogentin
Biperiden	Akineton
Chlorpromazine	Thorazine
Dicyclomine	Bentyl
Diphenhydramine	Benadryl
Disopyramide	Norpace
Doxepin	Sinequan, Adapin
Glycopyrrolate	Robinul
Imipramine	Tofranil
Loxapine	Loxitane
Maprotiline	Ludiomil
Mepenzolate	Cantil
Molindone	Moban
Nortriptyline	Aventyl
Procyclidine	Kemadrin
Propantheline	Pro-Banthine
Protriptyline	Vivactil
Thioridazine	Mellaril
Trihexyphenidyl	Artane
Trimipramine	Surmontil

Index

Organizations associated with mobility and mobility problems, 119-23
Orthostatic hypertension, balance and, 82, 84
Orthostatic hypotension, transfer and, 38
Osteoporotic compression fractures, transfer and, 40

P

Parker, D., 14
Parkinsonism, drugs for, 111, 112, 161
Patient's movement pattern, 24
Peripheral neuropathies, drugs associated with, 158
Perry, J., 65
Pill swapping, 107. *See also* Drugs
Posture, balance test and, 146-47. *See also* Standing posture
Presbycusis (high-frequency sound range loss), 93-94. *See also* Hearing loss
Presbyopia (old age blindness), 94-95. *See also* Vision loss
Pressure sores (decubitus ulcers)
  bed activity and, 14-15, 16
  bed making and, 133
  causes of, 125
    friction, 130
    pressure, 127-28
    moisture, 130
    shearing force, 128-30
  chair-bound patients and, 128
  costs of caring for patients with, 14, 125
  debridement and, 137
  dressing and wound care and, 135-40
  folk remedies (avoiding) and, 135
  myths and misconceptions concerning, 134
  nutrition and, 140-41

percentage of patients with, 125
physiologic approach to, 126
positioning to avoid, 15
prediction of, 126-27
prevention and, 126, 141-42
proper term for, 126
protective devices and, 131-34
screening for, 14-15, 16, 127, 128
risk factors for, 132
sitting and, 35
skin care and, 136, 139
stages of, 131
treatment of, 134-42
wheelchair use and, 128
Prone position (bed activity), 18
Protein binding, drugs and, 108
Psychological problems (confusion, fear, etc.) and balance problems, 82
Psychosocial area (drugs), 112
Ptophobia (fear of falling), 82. *See also* Falls

Q

Quad sets (balance exercise), 153

R

Range of motion decrease in elderly, 65
Range of motion exercises (sitting), 34
Response time build up (sensory loss), 104
Richter, R. R., 17, 37
Roger's Health Status Scale, 7, 8